Blue Juice

Blue Juice

Euthanasia in Veterinary Medicine

PATRICIA MORRIS

TEMPLE UNIVERSITY PRESS PHILADELPHIA

TEMPLE UNIVERSITY PRESS
Philadelphia, Pennsylvania 19122
www.temple.edu/tempress

Library of Congress Cataloging-in-Publication Data

Morris, Patricia (Patricia Hope), 1976–
   Blue juice : euthanasia in veterinary medicine / Patricia Morris.
      p. ; cm. — (Animals, culture, and society)
   Euthanasia in veterinary medicine
   Includes bibliographical references and index.
      ISBN 978-1-4399-0705-4 (cloth : alk. paper) —
   ISBN 978-1-4399-0706-1 (paper : alk. paper) —
   ISBN 978-1-4399-0707-8 (e-book)
      I. Title.   II. Title: Euthanasia in veterinary medicine.
III. Series: Animals, culture, and society.
      [DNLM: 1. Euthanasia, Animal.   2. Bonding, Human-Pet.
3. Pets—psychology.   4. Professional-Patient Relations.
SF 756.394]
      636.089'6029—dc23
                                                2011047604

Printed in the United States of America

102714P

Contents

Acknowledgments

My deepest gratitude goes to the many veterinarians who welcomed me into their world and then generously answered my many questions. I was fortunate to experience overwhelming kindness, enthusiasm, and encouragement from all the participants in this research project, but I am especially indebted to Carter Luke and Sharon Drellich. In addition, I thank my friend Dr. Elizabeth Lowe for introducing me to the world of veterinarians and for giving me the courage to choose a career I love. She is an amazingly dedicated veterinarian (and I have met many, so I can say this with confidence) and a tireless advocate for her patients and for all animals.

This book would not have been possible without the expert guidance of my esteemed mentors, Arnold Arluke and Clinton Sanders, whose work I greatly admire and borrow from heavily and who both offered detailed and thoughtful comments on several drafts along the way. The debt I owe Professor Arluke is in a class by itself. For many years, he has been a wonderful adviser and one of my strongest advocates in both my personal and professional life. Through his guidance and encouragement, the often daunting tasks of ethnographic work (gaining entry, dealing with sometimes reluctant participants, putting in long hours of field research, and analyzing lengthy interviews) gradually became a more comfortable process. I fully credit (and playfully blame) him for shaping me into the sociologist, scholar, teacher, and person that I am today. I only hope that I can inspire my students as he has inspired me.

Along with Professors Arluke and Sanders, Justin Betz, Silvia Dominguez, Jeremy Eggerman, Janet Francendese, Andrea Hill, Tom Koenig, Elizabeth Lowe, Amy Lubitow, and several anonymous reviewers generously sacrificed their limited free time to review parts (or all) of the unpolished early drafts of the manuscript. Their thoughtful comments greatly enhanced the finished product. It is impossible to sufficiently thank Jeremy for the emotional and technical support he provided during the final editing stages. In addition to taking out the trash and cooking dinner, he regularly spent whole weekends organizing references and tracking down missing information. Janet spent countless hours guiding me throughout the publishing process and overseeing the transition from proposal to finished manuscript. I am sincerely grateful to Janet and the entire editorial staff at both Temple University Press and Newgen for their professionalism, patience, dedication, and tireless attention to detail. I also gratefully acknowledge Northeastern University, Drury University, and the Charlotte W. Newcombe and Woodrow Wilson National Fellowship Foundations for their generous support of my research.

Other colleagues and friends have been tremendous assets in both work and play, including Makis Antzoulatos, Tammi Arford, Judy Brown, Michelle Creed, Dave Derossett, Meghan Doran, Mark Geiss, Trever Glode, Alan Klein, Alicia LaPolla, Jack Levin, Owen McLean, Lauren Nicoll, Gordana Rabrenovic, Kat Rickenbacker, Joanna Small, Stanislav Vysotsky, and Katie Yang. I am also grateful to my valued colleagues at Drury University: Jeanie Allen, Jana Bufkin, Valerie Eastman, Kathy Jester, Jennie Long, Vickie Luttrell, A. L. Marsteller, Patricia McEachern, Robin Miller, Jennie Silva-Brown, and Mary Utley. I especially thank Eric Madfis for his sympathy and support when I returned from long hours of emotionally draining fieldwork. I am also grateful to Andrea Hill for her clear-headed perspective on sociological issues, for her proofreading assistance, and for her friendship. If she had not cofounded the "zone of productivity," Chapter 1 would never have been written. Amy Lubitow helped with transcription, and she and Justin Betz contributed greatly to the analysis of data for Chapter 4. From the beginning, Justin calmly withstood my fits of anxiety and self-doubt and helped me see matters clearly. I am fortunate that he has been—and that he will always remain—such an important part of my life.

Over the many years of research and writing, I have benefited from extraordinary support and patience from my family, especially my dad, my mom, and my six younger siblings, Aimee, Laura Beth, Jessica, Matthew, Tiffany, and Joseph (as well as from each of my many precious nieces and nephews). My list of family supporters would not be complete without Steve Trenthem, Adam Logan, and Amanda, Susan, and Michael Spencer. I am also grateful to Jerry and Sherry Turner, April Turner, and Chris Przybyszew-ski for making me a part of their family and for encouraging me from my kindergarten days forward. I also acknowledge the loving friendships of Betsy Johnson, Liz Lowe, and Lauren Rolfe—all of whom remind me that family is as much created as it is inherited. I am forever indebted to everyone involved in the excitement, frustration, and rich rewards that this project has brought me—each of whom has helped me in ways that I cannot adequately put into words. I offer my heartfelt thanks to all.

Blue Juice

Introduction

Euthanasia in Veterinary Medicine

Euthanasia is different for today's vets. Today people have
varying relationships with their pets, but very often they will
see their pets as members of their family. They may relate to
euthanizing their pets as killing their child. . . . This is kind
of a new paradigm with regard to euthanasia. The old way of
doing things was, when a person wanted to euthanize their dog,
you would take it in the back and it gets euthanized. . . . The
client was really not involved in the process at all. We are really
getting away from that, but there are still veterinarians that do
that. There are still some veterinarians where it is a business
thing. You go up front and pay the money, and the dog goes in
the back and gets euthanized. It is not warm at all. Most people
now, however, want to be more *intimately* involved with
euthanasia. They want it to be a *nice* experience.

> —Forty-four-year-old veterinary professor
> in a lecture on euthanasia to his graduating seniors

As companion animals, or pets, increasingly become part of
American households and, for some, a valued part of the family, the termination of an animal's life has also become the
purview of veterinarians. Time and time again, small-animal veterinarians, like the professor in the opening quotation, explained to me how
euthanasia has changed. In today's veterinary offices, veterinarians and
their human clients share in the experience of an animal companion
being "put to sleep." For veterinarians, this event is routine, as they
may orchestrate it daily in their work. For many pet owners, having
made the agonizing decision to euthanize, it is a rare, highly emotional
experience.

Ask a typical American pet owner about his or her animal companion and
you will likely be told not only the species but also the breed, age, personality, and favorite foods, as well as how cute, smart, or brave the animal seems.

Such a response, although common today, would have astonished people a century ago, when animals rarely lived inside the house and certainly did not wear special holiday sweaters to pose for family portraits. Today people bond with their pets on various levels, considering them anything from annoying or costly accessories to valued family members. Perhaps at no time are these bonds more apparent than when pet owners face the decision of whether to end an animal's life. For some pet owners, simply anticipating that last trip they will make to the veterinarian with their beloved companions is stressful, and actually dealing with their pets' terminal illness, unexpected injury, or old age is an especially traumatic experience. Others have no such misgivings in similar circumstances; for them, the decision is straightforward and less emotionally wrenching. Whatever the mind-set of the owners, veterinarians must facilitate these life-and-death situations.

As a social scientist interested in medical sociology, death and dying, and human-animal relationships, I wanted to know more about how veterinarians deal with euthanasia and the interactions it entails. I spent a year and a half speaking with small-animal veterinarians and observing day-to-day activities in several veterinary hospitals. Being in treatment rooms with many veterinarians and clients as they made decisions or provided care gave me a bird's-eye view of the interactions between veterinary doctors and their human clients, animal patients, technicians, and colleagues. Although I often found my fieldwork emotionally upsetting and physically exhausting, research from a distance could not give me the access to the private and emotionally charged interactions between veterinarians and their clients that direct involvement could. Simply put, people reveal much more to an outsider willing to share in the ordinary day-to-day experiences than they do on a standardized questionnaire.[1]

Although this book focuses exclusively on the experiences of small-animal veterinarians, I had initially become interested in the study of euthanasia after hearing a fascinating story from a large-animal veterinarian. During his first month working for a busy large-animal practice, the young doctor was sent on a presumably routine checkup of a sick cow at a well-regarded client's dairy farm. Business with the cow concluded, the client, a rather burly farmer, inquired if he would mind euthanizing the family's pet chicken. Choking back a laugh, the novice feared he was the target of a hazing ritual or a practical joke. However, the family's earnest and somber demeanor told him this family had a special attachment to the chicken and wanted a peaceful death for their beloved companion. Rather than disappoint his new client and colleagues, the young veterinarian reluctantly agreed to euthanize the pet chicken.

In addition to a lack of confidence in his ability to deal with grieving clients, the novice veterinarian's reluctance to euthanize stemmed from a more practical concern—how to best euthanize a chicken. His training had indicated that cervical dislocation, or breaking the neck, would be the quickest and most humane method for the species, but he feared it would not *appear* peaceful or painless to the family. The veterinarian decided to instead use the more aesthetically pleasing method of intravenous barbiturate overdose, commonly used to euthanize pet animals, but he did not know the amount of solution to inject. After injecting the solution, and apprehensive that the animal might be only temporarily anesthetized, he created a pretext to get the family out of the room by suggesting that they gather a box and blanket for burial. In their absence he performed the cervical dislocation.

As he told me the story, his tone of voice and facial expressions strongly suggested that he saw the events of the chicken euthanasia as peculiar and harrowing and also somewhat comical. He exclaimed, "I actually had to 'euthanize' a family's dying chicken—if you can believe that! . . . What really got me is how attached this family was to this one chicken—like it was their dog or something." His astonished emphasis on *euthanize* led me to surmise that he did not typically think of the death of his patients as euthanasia. And he was clearly not accustomed to thinking of a chicken as a valued family pet.

I begin the book with the tale of a chicken euthanasia for two reasons. First, the anecdote points to how a client's regard for an animal shaped the interaction between the veterinarian and the client. A chicken's status as a valued family companion governed the method the veterinarian used to end this chicken's life. The story further demonstrates how veterinarians stage the death of animals for the benefit of their human clients. In fact, I found the efforts of veterinarians to create a good death for patients and an appearance of such for clients so compelling that I devote Chapter 2 to the subject.

Second, the chicken story reflects the complicated and shifting relationships between humans and animals. The *Wall Street Journal* published a series of articles on chickens' rise in popularity in urban neighborhoods.[2] People keep chickens for fresh eggs but also as companion animals, with some even becoming house pets. Several online forums address the emotional side of raising chickens and dealing with their death (see, for example, http://poultryone.com). Other people see chickens primarily as food, relating to their death in the same way the young veterinarian did to his poultry patient—"It's no big deal—it's *just* a chicken" (emphasis added). As this veterinarian's statement demonstrates, many do not understand the grief felt by enthusiasts over the loss of such a bird. Yet even though the young veterinarian was bewildered by the family's grief, he did his best to respect their relationship with the chicken.

The small-animal veterinarians in this book often go out of their way to convey to their clients that grief over the death of any animal is normal and legitimate. Consider the case of a young software engineer and his pet mouse, named Sam. Upon hearing that his companion would likely not survive, the young man was inconsolable. Behind closed doors, some staff members could not understand his attachment to a mouse and joked to each other, "This guy is nuts. He is crying about a mouse!" Though the veterinarian herself struggled to understand this client's emotional attachment to a mouse, she quickly chastised her staff: "That mouse meant a great deal to this guy, and if we in the veterinary profession think that his grief is strange, who else is going to understand what he is going through? It is our *job* to support his feelings about this mouse and make him feel like it is okay to cry over the death of a mouse."

When a human dies, most families are surrounded by nurturing friends and other family. But when a pet dies, families rarely receive the same attention. Although some friends and family may want to comfort loved ones after the death of a beloved animal, they may not fully understand or appreciate the loss. For example, the well-intentioned suggestion "You might feel better if you get another dog" can seem to some pet owners the same as "Don't worry. You can get a new spouse." Other, less sympathetic people may consider grieving for animals to be silly or overly sentimental and respond to the loss with an insensitive remark such as "It's *only* a cat. What's the big deal?"

Rather than deal with insensitivity or misunderstanding, some pet owners want to suppress, or at least hide, their emotions over the loss of an animal companion, but they often regard the veterinary office as a judgment-free place to express their grief. Although I observed some pet owners as they made seemingly callous decisions regarding the death of their animals, I also witnessed euthanasias in which extremely distraught owners asked to hold their companion animals during the process and spend time with the bodies afterward. I frequently observed such ends for the death of not just dogs and cats but also birds, mice, ferrets, hamsters, and an iguana.

Narratives on the death of patients in this book reveal the emotional role of modern companion-animal veterinarians in comforting bereaved pet owners. For example, as shown in the death of the mouse Sam, although the veterinarian was bewildered by her client's grief, she took him to the grieving room and offered sympathy. She even searched the Internet to find appropriately sized options for a casket or urn in case her client desired one. Concerned that many of their clients will not receive sufficient emotional support or sympathy from others for their loss, veterinarians told me that they often feel a special obligation to validate all of their clients' grief. For a sociologist, these emotion-laden encounters between veterinarians and their clients provide a rich context for examining how emotionality is managed in professional settings. The affective role veterinarians assume in comforting bereaved clients is the topic of Chapter 3.

To capture the breadth of encounters that unfold between clients, animals, and veterinarians regarding euthanasia, I consider the range and complexity of people's relationships with animals. For many social scientists, talking about *any* aspect of human-animal interaction requires a discussion of humans' ambiguous perceptions of other animals.[3] For example, some people may view an animal as a functional object, while others see it more as a companion subject. Some children enrolled in horseback riding lessons may see the horse as basically a vehicle, while others relate to it as a large pet.[4] People train dogs to fight to their death, race them for gambling purposes, leave them chained to fences in the backyard, breed them in puppy mills, train them for dog shows, take them on family vacations, buy them designer accessories, pamper them with spa treatments, or leave them substantial inheritances. Such wide-ranging treatment of horses and dogs provides just a few examples of the ambiguity inherent in our relationships with nonhuman animals.

Social scientists interested in human-animal relationships frequently note that animals play both utilitarian and affectional roles in many people's lives.[5] In other words, a person may regard different members of the same species as a subject or an object. As I discussed earlier, chickens are usually seen as functional objects (poultry to eat), but some people see them as sentient individuals (cherished pets). The dairy farming family in the pet chicken story raised most of their chickens for eggs and meat, but one chicken joined the family as a pet. Along similar lines, farm animals are property (commodities for profit), yet some farmers develop emotional connections to their cattle, pigs, and sheep. In her study of Scottish farmers, for example, Rhoda Wilkie found that farmers do not relate to their animals as simply property.[6] Indeed, as commodities, animals are seen as future meat and producers of dairy products, but farmers may also name, pamper, and feel affection for them. As one would expect, the emotional ambivalence inherent in these relationships is most troubling when it comes time to slaughter the animals.

While observing employees in animal-related workplaces, social scientists repeatedly find that occupational behavior reflects the ambiguity inherent in human-animal relationships. For example, in his studies of guide dog trainers, Sanders speculates that defining service dogs as both subjects and objects explains their simultaneous perception as equipment trained to serve, protect, and assist and as companions with whom one develops a shared emotional bond.[7] Other scholars bring to light similarly complicated relationships between workers and animals in a wide variety of settings, including biomedical laboratories,[8] primate labs,[9] animal shelters,[10] race tracks,[11] veterinary and medical schools,[12] and animal-cruelty law enforcement stations.[13]

Many scholars contend that these ambiguous perceptions and ambivalent emotions regarding nonhuman animals are fundamental aspects of human-animal interaction. For example, Hal Herzog playfully titled a recent book *Some We Love, Some We Hate, Some We Eat*, alluding to humans' inconsistent treatment of other animals.[14] Andrew Rowan argues that such attitudes are deeply entrenched in human society, calling it the "constant paradox."[15] Arnold Arluke and Clinton Sanders introduce the concept of a sociozoologic scale in part to explain such paradoxical treatment.[16] An animal's position on the scale determines whether as a society we worship, protect, segregate, or destroy those of its kind. Although positions along the scale vary considerably from culture to culture and change over time within any given culture, generally speaking, the more an animal is regarded as being like us, the less we will tolerate, ignore, or condone its mistreatment.

As medical providers to nonhuman animals, veterinarians are in a position that exemplifies the ambiguity inherent in human-animal relationships—they treat animals as both subjects (patients who deserve quality medical care) and objects (the client's property).[17] Thus, I was not at all surprised to see veterinary staff refer to an animal equally and interchangeably as a patient receiving care and as the owner's pet. Similarly, people who bring their animals into the veterinary hospital are as likely to be referred to as the pets' owners as they are the clients. In a similar way, throughout this book, I refer to those who pay for veterinary services as clients, owners, and caretakers and those who receive veterinary care as patients, companion animals, and pets.

Though most participants in my study use these terms interchangeably, many are sensitive to a budding debate in both the veterinary and animal rights communities. Some companion-animal veterinarians argue against the use of the terms *pet* and *owner* because they objectify animals in their care and, as a result, devalue the profession. Others, whether or not sympathetic to the argument, do not wish to make their terminology a political statement that might offend clients. Certain members of the multifaceted animal rights community contend that such words symbolize the oppression inherent in pet keeping. While I am aware of the ideological debates that surround these words, I use them largely for variety and because those I studied use them as commonplace designations.

Veterinarians encounter clients with widely disparate views and attitudes regarding animals in their charge. An animal's position along the continuum from valued subject (a patient deserving quality medical care) to functional object (the client's property) has clear implications for the kind of treatment it receives. For example, a client whose child has grown tired of the responsibility of taking care of a pet may request that the veterinarian euthanize a healthy, well-behaved animal. Yet pet owners who insist that the veterinarian carry out life-sustaining treatment or painful surgery on dying animals are just as common.

As subjects, companion animals provide valued emotional support to pet owners[18] who consider them cherished friends or even family members.[19] Some owners can conceive of circumstances in which they would choose to give a scarce drug to their pets rather than to a person outside the family.[20] These animals may receive hundreds or thousands of dollars' worth of veterinary care. According to the 2006 American Veterinary Medical Association (AVMA) national survey on pet ownership, U.S. households spent approximately $24.5 billion on unspecified veterinary care for more than seventy-two million dogs and nearly eighty-two million cats.[21] At one of the veterinary teaching hospitals featured in this book, a recently retired veterinarian recalled the time Elvis Presley chartered a plane to bring his companion animal to a state-of-the-art facility. Flying your dog from Memphis to Boston was extravagant in the 1960s and still is, but more and more of today's pet owners travel great distances to take their beloved companions to facilities offering the most sophisticated veterinary care available.

An article in the *New Yorker* in 2003 explored the question of how far Americans might go to prolong the health and comfort of their pets.[22] As it turns out, regardless of wealth, people are willing to devote considerable sums to the care and well-being of their companion. Some pet owners are willing to incur significant expense to save or extend the lives of their dying animals, demanding more high-tech care for diseases such as diabetes, heart disease, and cancer. Increasingly, animals receive advanced medical, dental, and surgical care, including dialysis, root canals, hip replacements, chemotherapy, cataract extractions, and even pacemakers. As a result, veterinarians can now become board-certified specialists in over thirty fields, including cardiology, radiology, ophthalmology, and oncology.

In addition to providing medical care to animal patients, veterinarians may also offer cosmetic and medically unnecessary services as requested by their human clients—for example, partial tail or ear removal required to meet breed standards or surgical amputation of a cat's claws to protect household items.[23] Regardless of whether clients requesting these services regard their animal as a family member, such surgeries relegate the animal to the status of an object by disregarding its distress and the potential for harm. For example, clipping ears or tail limits a canine's ability to communicate with other dogs, and loss of claws hinders a feline's ability to defend itself. Moreover, because some pet owners are unwilling to spend even minimal dollars on an animal they see as easily replaceable, veterinarians are asked to euthanize animals for non-life-threatening conditions. Some pet owners adopt animals for a very specific purpose, such as guard dog or jogging companion; if the animals become unable to perform the desired function, their owners may replace them. For example, although treatment may be available to ease the animal's discomfort, an arthritic dog might be put down, or euthanized, because the animal is no longer able to patrol the yard or keep up during the owner's evening jogs. Thus, though arthritis is not fatal to humans, it can be for non-human animals.

Legally, companion animals are property and can be euthanized for any rationale their owners devise. Although *euthanasia* can refer to ending the life of a human or a nonhuman animal, what qualifies as euthanasia for each group differs considerably. The word derives from the Greek *eu* ("good" or "well") and *thanatos* ("death"). For humans, calling a death *euthanasia* is restricted to circumstances of mercy killing, in which death is a welcome relief from prolonged pain and suffering. For nonhuman animals, a good death is defined not by motive but by method. In other words, so long as death is without pain and distress, animals are *euthanized* in animal shelters, veterinary offices, and research laboratories for the convenience and benefit of humans.

Traditionally, shelter workers referred to the death of animals in their care as *euthanasia* because they considered it a painless end to an otherwise cruel life of starving in the streets or being kept in cages for years. However, some in the sheltering community known as no-kill advocates argue that a focus on method without regard to rationale devalues the lives of animals.[24] Similar reasoning would never be used to justify the death of humans. Capital punishment, for example, no matter how painlessly performed, is not euthanasia. For no-kill shelter workers, the routine killing of unwanted, healthy animals should not be euphemistically referred to as *euthanasia*. They wish to apply the same standards for euthanasia to animals that are applied to humans.

Euthanasia is rarely a legal practice for physicians and remains controversial among practitioners for reasons whose elaboration is beyond the scope of this book.[25] Briefly stated, physicians opposed to legalized euthanasia argue that aiding in the death of patients violates the physician's professional oath to do no harm. They regard decisions related to euthanasia as too great a moral burden for physicians. Advocates of euthanasia, however, believe that patients should have the right to choose death to end their pain and suffering and that medical assistance is consistent with the physician's oath to serve the welfare and interests of the patient.

Physicians on both sides of the issue of legalized euthanasia share concerns about establishing safeguards and defining precisely what justifies ending suffering, which is necessary to prevent abuse by family members who stand to inherit money or avoid mistakes by hasty medical professionals.[26] Many physicians fear that, even with strong safeguards, legalized euthanasia could create a culture in which sick people feel obligated to choose euthanasia rather than impose financial burdens on their families. Physicians even grapple over the best terminology to describe their role in helping a person die—physician-assisted suicide, medically assisted dying, medicide (Kevorkian's term),[27] mercy killing, or terminal sedation. Debates aside, few physicians support ending a life that is not marked by severe, incurable suffering.[28]

Veterinarians euthanize patients with serious or incurable diseases, and they also must consider other reasons for euthanizing patients when death is clearly not in an animal's best interest. In this respect, euthanasia presents very different considerations for veterinarians than for physicians who treat humans. As I have suggested, pet owners have widely disparate views on the moral status of animals, ranging from assigning them significantly less to, at times, greater moral value than humans. Some owners request euthanasia for their healthy animals because of loud barking, damage to furniture or property, or failure to use the litter box. Even well-behaved animals can be euthanized because their owners move to an apartment with lease restrictions, develop an allergy, or no longer wish to care for the animal.

While such requests are fairly rare, veterinarians frequently must deal with more complicated dilemmas. Sometimes euthanasia of an elderly animal seems warranted if the increasing demands on the human caregiver become onerous. However, in some of these cases, the veterinarian might be sympathetic to a client's situation but unconvinced that the burden on the owner is great enough to justify the animal's death. Life-and-death decisions often have to be made on the basis of an owner's ability to pay for life-extending treatment. For example, an animal could recover completely with a $900 surgical fix, but the owner cannot pay for the surgery. When an alternative to euthanasia costs more than clients are willing or able to pay, veterinarians must decide if they are comfortable performing euthanasia.

Decisions regarding euthanasia of companion animals are rarely straightforward, and veterinarians and their clients must work together to make difficult choices. Pet owners have to decide how much time, energy, and money they can devote to care for their animals. Care for sick animals often has to do with where individuals choose to draw the line. What should be done when a hundred-pound, arthritic bullmastiff experiences increasing difficulty walking up and down stairs to the client's third-floor apartment? What about the diabetic cat who requires daily shots? Should the veterinarian continue sustaining the life of a sick or severely injured animal with only a small chance of survival? Veterinarians must decide for themselves when killing an animal is justifiable and whether they can ethically refuse a client's request to perform euthanasia or continue life-sustaining treatment.

In this book I do not seek answers to such philosophical questions. Though I recognize that the morality of human behavior is of great importance to society and the veterinary profession, several prominent philosophers have already written books specifically for veterinarians to help them reflect on such weighty questions.[29] As a social scientist, I am interested in the subfield of descriptive ethics, which seeks to uncover people's moral beliefs and behaviors. Rather than determine the correctness or consistency of such beliefs, I examine what people think and do when confronting moral quandaries. From a sociologically informed perspective, this book provides an account of veterinarians' hands-on experience negotiating with clients and deciding when ending an animal's life is ethically appropriate.

My study's participants repeatedly described the practice of euthanasia to me as both "the best and worst part of [their] job." On one hand, euthanasias were fraught with ethical dilemmas and frustrations that forced them to develop emotionally protective strategies. Some euthanasias were so psychologically draining that veterinarians were hard pressed to perform this dirty aspect of their job. On the other hand, participants described euthanasia experiences as professionally rewarding and personally gratifying. For many, being good at euthanasia and helping pet owners through the grieving process formed an important part of their identity as accomplished veterinarians. Perhaps ironically, many veterinarians expressed a surprisingly similar version of the following sentiment: "You can tell a lot about a veterinarian by the way he or she handles euthanasia. How you end your patient's life can be just as important as healing the patient."

Trained and committed to saving animals and improving their lives, veterinarians can suddenly find their role changing from doing all they can to prolong an animal's life to ending it. While euthanasia is not always an emotionally taxing act, the types of situations that provoke stress for individual veterinarians depend greatly on their personal values and attitudes. Given the wide range of beliefs and values regarding the proper treatment of animals, all veterinarians will likely confront disagreement with some clients when negotiating life-and-death outcomes for their patients. Veterinarians take a professional oath to serve both the animal patient and the human client, and many experience significant moral stress when they perceive a conflict between these obligations.[30] Trying to reconcile their moral views about animals with those of their clients, most veterinarians regularly face taxing moral quandaries related to euthanasia.

When veterinarians and their clients do not share the same moral values regarding animals, they must work together to determine when euthanasia is a reasonable choice. At times a veterinarian may persuade clients to take a different course, but this process is often tiring and frustrating. For example, unlike in most doctor-patient interactions, frank discussions of cost of care as it relates to life-and-death issues are common in veterinarian-client relationships.[31] Talking about financing an animal's care can make veterinarians feel less like doctors and more like car mechanics, and veterinary staff often make light of these negotiations with clients by jokingly comparing their actions to those of used-car salesmen. But selling every client on the medically ideal but expensive Cadillac plan is not realistic. Thus veterinarians must offer concessions—potentially at a patient's expense—by presenting clients with more-affordable treatment, from the practical Volvo plan all the way down to the unreliable (and perhaps deadly) Ford Pinto plan.

Negotiations that involve bargaining with owners over treatment costs to avoid euthanasia are particularly unsavory for most veterinarians and can be especially troubling for novices. As participants gained experience in clinical settings, they almost universally began to cynically express their frustration with such disappointing realities of veterinary practice. For example, when reflecting on their patients as a whole, most made note of an upsetting paradox:

> Money is a tricky thing in veterinary medicine. . . . There is such a thing as a client having too much money and [one having] too little money. On one hand, you have people who put their animal down for treatable procedures or curable conditions. On the other hand, you have people who spend money to keep patients alive when it is not in the best interest of the animal. You can see how the financial status of the owner can screw a patient. . . . Veterinary medicine has a lot to do with money.

After facing such disparities in resources and willingness to pay for an animal's care, novices quickly learned that both types of negotiations often end in disappointing outcomes for the veterinarian.

Most veterinarians, regardless of their level of experience, report at least some emotional difficulty with performing euthanasia when they are not persuaded by the rationale for an animal's death; some even describe feeling they are killers or murderers at such times. Sometimes humor eases or masks a veterinarian's discomfort in dealing with difficult cases. Veterinarians and their assistants often mock clients who choose euthanasia for reasons staff consider trivial or illegitimate. For example, families suspected of spending thousands of dollars on designer dog collars or recreational activities are scoffed at behind closed doors for claiming that they are unable or unwilling to pay a relatively small amount for their animals' care: "We joke about the nerve of some owners coming in here wearing expensive jewelry, but instead we have to kill their animal. We joke when they drive away in a brand-new Mercedes or have a big fat diamond on their hand and they are not willing to fork over five hundred bucks for their pet. We can't really say it to their faces so we size them up when they leave."

For many veterinarians the only request worse than killing an animal for trivial reasons is sustaining the life of an animal when cure or even comfort is not possible. Veterinarians believe people desire to keep animals alive in many of these cases, not because it is good for the animal, but because it is too difficult to make the decision to end the life of a beloved companion animal. Here, veterinarians and their staff are torn between their obligation to provide the life-sustaining measures the client demands and their own desire to end the patient's suffering. Many participants in my study reported that one of the most difficult aspects of their job was to have to convince someone it was time to let go of a dying pet.

In these cases veterinarians and their staff would wryly joke about euthanizing the patient by filling their syringes with "blue juice," an insider's term for the barbiturate solution used to cause the death of veterinary patients. This solution is often called blue juice or pink juice because of the dye used as a safety precaution to indicate the deadly concentration of barbiturate.[32] *Blue juice* was the slang used most often when veterinarians and their staff expressed frustration with difficult cases in which they could do little to improve the patient's condition but the client insisted that treatment continue. For example, a veterinarian would joke to a colleague, "I sure wish I could slip this poor fellow the blue juice." In support, the colleague would sarcastically ask if the patient might want to eat some chocolate cake (a treat that dogs often enjoy but can be toxic to them). This kind of humor not only communicates to fellow insiders that the decisions of clients are not favored but also provides a way for frustrated veterinarians to let off steam.

Recognizing that outsiders might be shocked or uncomfortable when first exposed to such terms, I use the slang term *blue juice* in the title of this book with some trepidation. One veterinary insider respectfully suggested I change the title to "Veterinary Euthanasia: The Art, Agony, and Science of Saying Good-bye." Naturally, I am concerned that some might misinterpret my study's participants as being disrespectful to patients and unsympathetic to clients. Yet to categorize veterinarians who use dark humor as unsympathetic toward clients or unconcerned with patients in their care would be a regrettable mistake. Such an assessment of veterinarians is no more fair—or accurate—than saying the same of physicians who use similar gallows humor in their work. More importantly, it is woefully inaccurate. The veterinarians whose lives I humbly attempt to represent in the following pages earned my sincerest admiration and respect for their patience, dedication, and compassion for both their human clients and the animals in their care.

Incorporating the slang term *blue juice* in the title is important to me because I believe it helps capture the complex and dynamic nature of veterinary euthanasia. Early in their careers veterinarians learn to adjust to the frequency with which they are called on to kill animals, but many waver in their feelings about euthanasia. On one hand, ending patients' intense pain and distress can be a great relief to veterinarians and their human clients. On the other hand—even when the patient is suffering considerably—ending the life of a patient can place a tremendous emotional burden on the veterinarian.

A more sedate, less charged title for this book, one distanced from insider language, would oversimplify the multifaceted reality that I found. Instead, I suggest that much can be gained from exploring the complex and ambiguous nature of veterinarians' experience with the practice of euthanasia. One is unlikely to find a veterinarian who accepts *no* reason for ending an animal's life, but one is equally unlikely to find one who *never* suffers conflict in relation to his or her role in euthanasia. The truth is that veterinarians are often hesitant to kill but resigned to the necessity of euthanasia in their work. They experience a wide variety of emotions related to euthanasia, including anger, apathy, intense distress, and great relief. Although a particularly salient emotion-management technique, humor is but one method of many outlined in Chapter 5 that veterinarians use to cope with these feelings.

The use of gallows humor and dark jargon in the workplace is certainly not unique to veterinary professionals; it is also found among many occupational groups that regularly deal with death-related experiences, including paramedics[33] and police officers,[34] firefighters,[35] nurses,[36] and medical doctors.[37] In all these occupations, sharing coded-language humor allows insiders to communicate strong emotions and, at times, soften tragedy. Scholars argue that gallows humor that disparages and depersonalizes death lessens the psychological impact of the experience and creates enough emotional distance for workers to mediate death-related experiences.[38] Ideally, this humor allows workers to create an emotionally safe distance but not entirely detach themselves from the situation.

Away from patients, physicians sometimes use humorous or sardonic expressions to describe death or dying, such as "circling the drain," "croaked," "kicked the bucket," "pushing up daisies," "bit the dust," or "bought the farm."[39] Though veterinarians also use these dark euphemisms, they have unique terms to describe the death of their patients, such as an animal "went paws up," "was given the *go-go juice*," or "was given the blue juice." We all use euphemistic language, although not as dark, to distance ourselves from the unpleasant realities related to death. For example, we often replace *dead* with "passed away," "no longer with us," "gone to a better place," or "departed." *Euthanasia* itself is used, at least partly, because people are uncomfortable with the term *killing*. While laboratory animals are "sacrificed,"[40] a companion animal is "euthanized," "sent to doggie heaven," "put down," or "put to sleep."

Although dark or gallows humor is an important tool for creating distance from emotionally troubling aspects of some activities, researchers acknowledge that too much of it can tip the delicate balance between distance and connection.[41] The problem occurs when a physician or veterinarian becomes emotionally overburdened, or burned out. At this point, humor is less a tool and more an indication that the medical professional has lost touch with the patient and sees only the disease. In these situations, dark humor can exacerbate a veterinarian's impatience, anger, and cynicism rather than help maintain emotional connections to patients. Ideally, humor allows workers to distance themselves from the anxiety associated with death-related tasks yet maintain emotional connection to those they are charged with helping.

Often companion-animal veterinarians must deal with not only the death of their patients but also emotionally distraught owners who wish to be involved in the death process. In researching this book I became captivated by euthanasias that resemble pseudofunerals. Veterinarians even describe their role in euthanasia as similar to that of a funeral director orchestrating rituals for pet owners. They often invite clients to bring friends and family members to be present during the euthanasia and to spend some time saying good-bye to the animal. Clients whose animals died during treatment are invited to postdeath viewings of their animals' remains in private rooms. The veterinarian may discuss with pet owners the pros and cons of burial versus cremation and even help them choose an urn or handcrafted wooden pet casket for an animal's remains. If an owner wishes to take the animal's body home for burial, the veterinarian may place the body in a coffin-shaped cardboard box. Many veterinary clinics have created special spaces designed specifically for euthanasia that resemble rooms one might see in funeral homes, with couches, wall decorations, and even fresh flowers.

Part of this book is therefore about Americans' relationship with animals as revealed in the death of their pets. The place of pets in American families is changing. Companion animals are increasingly included in the rituals of everyday family life. Pet owners include animals in family portraits, write letters in pets' voices, dress them in Halloween costumes, or celebrate their birthdays. Scholars interested in the role of the pet in the modern American family report that many people view animals as unique, emotional, reciprocating, and thoughtful friends or family members.[42] Considered on a par with familial relationships, pet ownership may explain why some people resist evacuating natural disaster areas.[43] Indeed, some people experience greater bonds with animals than they do with humans.[44] Given the emotional significance of modern animal companions,[45] their deaths have increasingly become significant stressors in the lives of pet owners.[46]

The study of euthanasia as practiced in veterinary medicine may provide answers to some larger and more human questions. Physicians and philosophers have long pondered, for example, how physicians would reconcile being both protectors of life and dispensers of death if euthanasia were legal for humans. By defining how veterinarians think, feel, and act regarding this aspect of their work, we see how direct involvement in the death of patients informs a doctor's identity. The experience of veterinarians may theoretically offer fresh insights into the practice of euthanasia in human medicine. What is missing from the larger conversation is the potential for physicians and veterinarians to learn valuable lessons from one another.

Although scholars in the public debate seldom consider veterinary professionals, these professionals have extensive practical experience with euthanasia. Without having to rely on hypothetical situations, those studying veterinary euthanasia may provide yet-unexplored insight related to end-of-life care in the medical profession. Every year a new cohort of young veterinarians, entering the workforce after graduation, must consider when euthanasia is justified, how best to achieve a good death for their patients, and how to make sense of their role in that death. Long-standing debates in human medicine over end-of-life care and euthanasia rarely consider how enhanced knowledge of animal euthanasia might shed light on the practice for humans. This book provides the baseline for comparisons and, on its own, is an important beginning to an exploration of euthanasia in practice.

For social scientists, the study of veterinary euthanasia provides a unique lens through which to study many important topics, including professional socialization, emotion management, and death and dying, as well as relationships between practitioners and patients or clients in a medical-care system that is ethically complex. Ethnographers have intensely observed the work worlds of doctors, nurses, lawyers, police, firefighters, salespeople, morticians, prostitutes, waitresses, corporate leaders, and even obituary writers, among countless others.[47] Yet a relative dearth of scholarly attention is given to the attitudes and actions of veterinarians.[48] Literature on professional work regarding death and dying typically focuses on doctors, nurses, hospice workers, pathologists, police, coroners, and funeral directors,[49] but the role of veterinarians in the death of their patients has been the focus of little empirical study.

Of course, many biographical accounts and personal memoirs of a day in the life of a veterinarian have been written by or about practitioners[50] and even animal hospitals.[51] James Herriot's book *All Creatures Great and Small* was so popular that the BBC made it the basis for a television series.[52] Though these accounts provide interesting anecdotes about veterinary practice, their authors do not systematically collect data or provide scholarly analysis. Interest in the scientific study of veterinarians has increased among social scientists.[53] Yet relatively few scholarly works are dedicated to the veterinary profession, and even fewer focus on issues of death and dying within the profession.[54] This book seeks to address such deficiencies in the study of veterinary medicine.

This book captures the drama, paradoxes, and often complicated interactions between small-animal veterinarians and pet owners contemplating life-and-death decisions for their companions. The subject matter and approach of the book are unique, as is the scope of what is covered—everything from telling owners bad news about their pets' conditions, to negotiating the many possible outcomes (including euthanasia), to handling the death of animals. As I demonstrate in Chapter 1, reaching a decision about when to end an animal's life is often a carefully negotiated process between the pet owner and the veterinarian. An owner might believe, for example, that a three-legged dog or a one-eyed cat would suffer and that she or he would be cruelly condemning the animal to a miserable life. Veterinarians who disagree sometimes change a client's mind by arguing, "I guarantee it will be more traumatic for you to lose a limb or an eye than it will be for your dog. An animal will not experience the social aspects. Most animals do just fine three legged or one eyed and they don't seem to mind it much." While some disagreements are easily dispatched, others require considerable effort for veterinarians and their clients to resolve. In some circumstances, amicable solutions to disagreements cannot be reached, and in very rare cases, law enforcement may be called in to preside over disputes.

Chapter 2 describes the efforts of veterinarians to create good deaths for their animal patients and a good last memory for their human clients. After a decision has been made to euthanize an animal, the veterinarian must direct the physical process, from the actual killing of the animal to dealing with its remains. Inviting witnesses to the death process poses new challenges, as veterinarians must now be concerned with managing clients' impressions of the death. The goal of a good euthanasia is a gentle slipping into death, which looks like an animal is quietly and painlessly falling asleep; however, despite the veterinarian's best efforts, this goal is not always accomplished. Chapter 2 captures the complicated ways veterinarians, attuned to all the opportunities for error and failure, direct each euthanasia drama and change the sterile medical environment into a personalized and intimate one. A good euthanasia, although precarious, can be deeply rewarding for the veterinarian and satisfying for the owner.

In Chapter 3, I take the reader into these very private moments that unfold between human clients, their animals, and veterinarians. Today's veterinarians face a new paradigm in which owners desire to be more intimately involved in the death of their pets—often displaying intense emotions. Veterinarians carefully manage such emotions for both instrumental and expressive ends. When a patient's life hangs in the balance, they help clients manage guilt and grief so clients can make timely decisions. After a client makes the difficult decision to euthanize a companion animal, the veterinarian's goals change from facilitating medical decisions to helping the client deal with the death of the animal. Recognizing the intense feelings of grief, pain, and sorrow resulting from the death of a pet, veterinarians help grieving clients resolve feelings of guilt they might have and offer them comfort and counsel.

Chapters 4 and 5 concern the difficulties of euthanasia for the veterinary practitioner from the points of view of the seasoned professional and the rookie veterinarian fresh out of school. By following an entire cohort of interns through their first year in practice, I was able to note the stressors unique to beginning practitioners who felt unprepared and even shocked by some realities of the job that challenged their idealistic expectations. By shadowing residents and board-certified specialists throughout the workday, I learned about the euthanasia-related stressors that continue after years of experience. Together, these two chapters show that novices eventually resolve some of their frustrations regarding the practice of euthanasia, while other related stressors prove to be especially difficult to manage—even for veterinarians with years of experience.

The Conclusion considers the myriad ways the practice of euthanasia highlights significant changes and controversies in veterinary medicine and in human-animal relationships. For example, as a result of the strengthening bonds between people and their companion animals, many small-animal veterinarians are revising the business of professional veterinary service to include not only maintaining the health and well-being of animals but also attending to the emotional needs of their clients. While some veterinarians consider this new role of offering comfort and counsel to clients to be outside their domain of knowledge, experience, and responsibility, others embrace the role. For those who embrace it, being good at dealing with owners' emotions has little to do with their professional training, yet they consider it an important part of their job.

As I show in the chapters that follow, each aspect of euthanasia reflects deep and unresolved tensions inherent in human-animal relationships that derive from treating animals simultaneously as subjects and objects, patients and property. Because animals exist somewhere between the categories of subject-patient and object-property, veterinarians encounter a wide variety of mixed and uncertain attitudes regarding animals from their colleagues and clients. While many young students today entering veterinary schools see animals as having a moral status closer to that of humans, much of the public and others in the profession do not share this perspective. In the process of becoming full-fledged veterinarians, these novices will not find it easy to balance their allegiance to clients, patients, and colleagues. In this nexus of multiple moral standpoints—exactly at the moment when issues of life and death are being decided—how do practitioners weigh the needs of their clients and their patients? This book considers that question.

Negotiating Death

Managing Disagreement with Pet Owners

D uring the course of my research, I was invited to attend a one-day seminar on euthanasia required of third-year students at my local veterinary college. Though truly grateful for the opportunity to sit in on the day's events, I must admit that an early morning discussion of the pharmacological effects of euthanasia drugs on biological systems was not how I was hoping to start my day. While I acknowledge that this subject is important to veterinarians, I still wished I had overslept. I began to perk up when the lectures turned to an analysis of different methods for providing animals a painless death given their species, breed, and particular illness. However, after lunch, I was positively thrilled when the professor opened her lecture by recalling a time one of her clients asked if, in the event of his death, she would euthanize his pet.

Upon his demise, the client wanted the veterinarian to euthanize his then eight-year-old German shepherd so the animal could be buried with him. The vet reluctantly agreed, in part because she thought her client might be joking but also because she did not believe that the man would die before his dog. Unfortunately, the client did die, and he was serious about his request. She now had to decide if she could keep her previous agreement with the client. In the end, she decided to honor her promise. Fortunately, her conscience was relieved by the fact that the dog was now twelve years old and had hip dysplasia and arthritis, serious conditions that helped her justify euthanasia at that time. However, the case forced her to think earnestly about what she might have done if the animal had been in better health and how she would manage such requests in the future.

The instructor surveyed the class, asking students how they felt about such a request and how they thought they might have negotiated a similar situation. Next, she presented more hypothetical questions for her students' consideration. Under what circumstances is it morally and ethically acceptable to euthanize an animal? Do clients have the right to ask the veterinarian to euthanize their animal regardless of its health? Would there be a justifiable difference between euthanizing a healthy (but aggressive) animal as opposed to a sick (but treatable) animal whose owner cannot afford the necessary surgery? Can veterinarians refuse extreme life-saving measures for animals they see as seriously suffering?

The instructor's probing hypothetical questions initiated frenzied ethical debates. After allowing the debates to continue for some time, the instructor proposed that sticking to one's ethical ideals may be more challenging in reality than students thought. The professor argued, and research suggests, that real-life and hypothetical dilemmas may elicit different responses.[1] The instructor asked her students to consider how they would act when a client asked them to do something their gut told them was wrong. Turning to one student who had earlier said that keeping animals on a ventilator was cruel, she asked, "How exactly do you *politely* tell a client that you think keeping their terminally ill companion on a ventilator is *cruel*?" She inquired, "How can you *convince* your elderly client that placing the cat in a shelter is a better alternative when he strongly believes that his cat loves him so much that she simply couldn't survive without him?" The professor continued, "How would you *negotiate* with the client that doesn't have the funds for treating their animal's condition but can't bear the thought of their pet 'suffering' in a shelter?"

Discussing Death with Clients

Though previous studies have gathered information on the moral orientation and general moral reasoning of practicing veterinarians,[2] like the veterinary professor, I wanted to know how my study participants resolved real life-and-death disagreements with clients. As it turns out, clients and veterinarians often come to mutually agreed on decisions; however, negotiations are substantially complicated if the veterinarian disagrees with client requests. When veterinarians are unwilling to carry out client requests, they assume an advocacy role for their patient. Sometimes disagreements are easily resolved, but at other times negotiations between veterinarians and clients become difficult. The purpose of this chapter is twofold: outline the common types of life-and-death disagreements veterinarians have with clients and discuss how veterinarians manage such disagreements.

In the beginning of my research, I naively thought I could simply gather a set of universally accepted guidelines regarding what constitutes a legitimate rationale for euthanasia. As it turns out, this is a difficult, if not downright impossible, task. First, my study participants vehemently fought my best efforts to uncover the standards they use for deciding when euthanasia is legitimate. They repeatedly stressed that they do not rely on a magic formula. Instead, because each case involves a unique combination of factors, their decision making is often case by case.

Moreover, although veterinarians may agree on the worthiness of a particular rationale for euthanasia, their criteria to establish legitimacy for such a claim varied from veterinarian to veterinarian. For example, most participants agreed that it is right to euthanize an animal whose quality of life is so impaired by disease or injury that it is inhumane to keep it alive, but they often disagreed on when this point is reached. In other words, the patient's quality of life is nearly universally considered the most legitimate rationale for euthanasia,[3] but there are no universally defined criteria to determine when an animal has a poor enough quality of life to justify euthanasia.

Veterinarians consider factors outside the animal's quality of life to be acceptable, although considerably less legitimate, reasons to euthanize. For example, veterinarians believe it important to weigh the odds of a successful outcome for the patient against an expensive treatment plan. Similarly, veterinarians disagree about how to draw such boundaries. For some, almost any cost the owner cannot afford, no matter how small, justifies euthanasia. For others, euthanizing an otherwise healthy animal with a good prognosis (e.g., a broken leg) because of the owner's inability to pay for reasonable treatment is unacceptable.

Despite participants' best efforts to avoid my questions regarding standards for legitimacy, I was able to uncover key aspects of their decision-making process. These factors typically included diagnosis and prognosis, quality of life, current symptom burden (stress, pain, and suffering), risk-benefit analysis of the proposed intervention, treatment financial cost, patient's past response to treatment interventions, species characteristics and life span, and treatment burden for the owner. For most participants, any one of these could constitute legitimate rationale for euthanasia. Again, the tricky part was getting them to agree on either the exact combination of factors or when one factor was severe enough to justify euthanasia. For instance, though many veterinarians support euthanasia of animals that present an obvious danger to society, they often disagree on when a pet's behavior has become risky, vicious, or unmanageable enough.

When several of the previously listed key factors are considered problematic enough, veterinarians have no dilemma about the need for euthanasia. For instance, Dr. Green described a clear-cut case for her as "a patient that has metastatic cancer and is geriatric with several comorbid conditions like heart disease and renal failure. . . . I always say any one of [those] alone may be manageable, but all of them together make Fluffy's prognosis really bad. I don't need a whole lot of conference to be okay with that decision." Patients who were old and infirm or suffering from severe illness or injury were generally considered the most legitimate cases for euthanasia.

One easily negotiated example involved two of Dr. Hill's favorite clients and their twelve-year-old Great Dane, Duke, who was unable to eat without a feeding tube because of a serious medical condition known as megaesophagus. As I understand the condition, the esophagus becomes so enlarged that it is unable to push swallowed food into the stomach, resulting in frequent vomiting and, unfortunately for Duke, chronic pneumonia. Even though less than 35 percent of patients recover from aspiration pneumonia, Duke's owners spent more than $3,000 in hopes of his living another year. Despite the owners' dedication and commitment to treating Duke, his condition remained poor. Thus, considering his poor quality of life, older age, difficult medical condition, and poor response to treatment, Dr. Hill easily supported her clients' decision to euthanize.

Ethically gray cases that balance uncertain health outcomes against a treatment's known adverse effects do not pose difficulties for most veterinarians, because they conclude that it is equally legitimate to treat or euthanize the animal. For example, many participants considered a diagnosis of hemoabdomen a gray issue because it is a potentially life-threatening condition that requires surgery to remove a bleeding tumor. An ultrasound and chest radiograph[4] can determine if the tumor has spread to the liver and lungs, indicating malignancy. If it has not spread, owners can proceed with surgery and hope the tumor is benign. If benign, prognosis is excellent for a full recovery; however, if it is malignant, survival time is much less optimistic. As one veterinarian put it, "There was a one in four chance that the surgery alone would fix the problem, but surgery is expensive. They may euthanize their animal because it is 4 to 5,000 dollars on a bet. It may be totally treatable, but it may be cancer, [and] then the dog would have maybe three months without chemo and six to eight months with chemo." In these types of gray-area prognoses, most participants were equally comfortable with euthanasia or surgical intervention.

Financial Issues

Though veterinarians accept the reality that finances play an important role in treatment decisions, they prefer that finances not be the primary factor in the decision to euthanize animals. Participants often reported that euthanizing for mostly financial concerns felt dirty or unsavory; when decisions were completely separated from finances, euthanizing felt clean and even comfortable: "It sometimes feels great when it has nothing to do with money, and no amount of money is going to make this any better for the cat. You can tell owners that, even if they were Bill Gates, . . . nothing can be done to save their cat—nice and clean."

Decisions based primarily on finances are not always problematic for veterinarians. When participants knew that their clients could not afford costly treatment, financially based decisions were more palatable to them. Moreover, high treatment costs are often associated with animal-related concerns (e.g., poor quality of life, potentially painful treatments, poor prognosis, or uncertain recovery). In other words, when treatment is costly for financial reasons or other patient-related factors that helps the veterinarian favor euthanasia.

However, financially based considerations for euthanasia may come up even when the animal's condition is far from life threatening. Some pet owners adopt animals without considering their financial commitment for a pet's medical needs, and many have unrealistic expectations about veterinary costs. In such cases owners may choose euthanasia because they cannot afford even minimal treatment costs for animals whose prognosis is excellent: "Sometimes pretty treatable diseases become untreatable when the owner can't pay for it. That sucks, but it happens."

At the other extreme are pet owners who are able to afford reasonable treatment options but who still want to euthanize their sick pet: "There are also people who have the money but won't spend a dime to fix a good prognosis." Dr. Cope, who practices in a wealthy neighborhood in California, describes such a case:

> The case was a [urinary] blocked cat, and I went round and round and round with this guy for almost two hours, and he finally signed the cat over to me, and we found him a new home after fixing him up. But [the client] was a jerk. He was cussing and swearing and calling us thieves because he thought we were charging too much. I finally got it through his head that we were not going to kill this cat because it is blocked. We don't kill cats because they can't pee. It is fixable.

Participants who worked in less affluent neighborhoods had similar stories of frustration, and they often drew the line for what they considered reasonable expenses far earlier than Dr. Cope. Regardless of the general socioeconomic status of their clientele, when treatment costs are deemed reasonable for the owner, veterinarians are hesitant to euthanize:

> Sometimes what we are asking is not that much, and we have done all we can to lower the costs so we are not getting paid what we deserve, and they still want to euthanize. It is terrible to feel like you are willing to sacrifice more for their animal than they are. If they truly just don't have the money and they have to choose between feeding their kids and treating their animal, that is different. . . . The financial [cases] where they are not that sick but the owner just won't make the sacrifice and cough up the money are the worst. It is fucking annoying when they drive up here in their Lexus or their Mercedes and they won't pay the eight hundred bucks it would take to totally fix their animal.

Assessing an owner's willingness to spend money on the animal is an important part of veterinary negotiation,[5] which can get complicated when euthanasia decisions are related exclusively to financial costs.

Behavioral Issues

Clients may request euthanasia for animals that are healthy but have certain behavioral issues (e.g., aggression, urinating outside litter box, chewing or scratching furniture, or excessive barking). Of all the problematic behavioral issues, veterinarians considered aggression the most legitimate reason to euthanize. Yet when clients presented aggressive animals for euthanasia, negotiation was not always straightforward. For instance, a veterinarian might disagree with an owner's definition of aggression: "I had a guy who came to euthanize his dog because he said that it was biting, so we went more in depth with it. . . . [I]f he [had] said to me that his animal bit his child, then I would be more accepting of that as a legitimate reason, but he said that the dog would chase the kids and nip at their feet, so then I was not okay with it." Participants disliked euthanizing "dangerous" animals when they could not gather enough evidence to establish that the animal was aggressive and likely to cause injury to another animal or a human.

Veterinarians were hesitant to honor requests for euthanasia for behavioral reasons they considered minor or tolerable nuisances, such as barking, acting too energetic, or scratching the furniture. However, they made exceptions if the behavior rendered the animal unadoptable (i.e., soiling the house): "If they won't quit peeing in the house, what are you going to do? They are not adoptable because nobody wants an animal to pee all over their house. Have you ever lived with a cat that keeps peeing on your couch? It is horrible." Though sympathetic to client frustration, many participants encouraged owners to make significant efforts to change the animal's behavior before they would agree to euthanasia: "If they eliminated all possible medical causes and they tried behavioral management techniques, I am okay with euthanizing the animal." Participants sometimes disagreed with an owner's request for euthanasia because they believed that the client did not try hard enough to solve the behavioral problem.

Treatment Burden

Clients may request euthanasia for an animal because they are not able or willing to care for the animal at home. Veterinarians often abhor euthanizing animals whose diagnosis is considered treatable, manageable, or even reversible, but when pets need substantial care at home they often agree to euthanasia because of demands on the pet owner. Dr. Stone, for example, easily supported an owner's decision to euthanize his 150-pound mastiff who was unable to walk on the grounds that rehabilitation posed a legitimate burden to the owner: "Even if he can be treated surgically, the six to eight weeks of home management can be very difficult even for small dogs. Dogs his size get a much worse prognosis just being big. . . . If he can't pee on his own, they [the clients] may have to learn how to pass a urinary catheter, and he may get urinary infections, and he will just shit all over the floor. It is really messy. They will have to carry him everywhere, and he may get bedsores too. It is a lot to take on."

However, veterinarians detest requests for euthanasia when they cannot see the burden on clients as serious enough to justify euthanasia. For example, Dr. Turner described a time when she was disappointed in her client's commitment to the health and well-being of his pet:

> I brought the guy into the room; the cat was a twelve-year-old Siamese, and he had diarrhea, and the owner said, "I can't keep up with all this diarrhea." "So you want to euthanize him because he's having diarrhea? Let's have a look at him." Maybe he's debilitated and has GI [gastrointestinal] lymphoma and is dehydrated and dying, so then I'd say, "Okay, let's go ahead and euthanize." But this cat was bright eyed,

beautiful coat, healthy appetite. He was walking and curious, exploring around. I know it is hard to deal with this, but we should see if
there is a treatment first.

Sometimes owners choose to euthanize their older animal because they have
other, competing responsibilities. For example, caring for young children may
prevent owners from giving the extra care and support their animal needs.

The veterinarian may believe an owner is not making enough effort to
solve a potentially minor, or easily fixable, health condition:

Yesterday I had a case of hyperthyroid. . . . That's something fixable.
It is giving a few pills, and for a minor inconvenience to you, your cat
could've lived, and she [the owner] just didn't want to hear it. I still
can't figure out what was wrong with that owner. She just refused.
Sometimes they just want it to be something simple [that] you just
give a pill to once and then it's fixed, and otherwise they don't want
to deal with it.

Owners may believe they could not give their pill-resistant cat daily medications or their diabetic dog insulin shots, or they may simply not want
the inconvenience. The veterinarian may oppose these types of euthanasia
requests, seeing the necessary tasks to care for the animal as too minor to
justify euthanasia.

Euthanasia of Healthy Animals

Animals with no health or behavioral problems are sometimes brought in for
euthanasia. Pet owners moving to a place that does not allow animals may
request that their pet be euthanized. Elderly people may not be allowed to
take pets into institutional housing, or perhaps they are no longer able to care
for their otherwise healthy animal. Owners may wish to euthanize because
they had unrealistic expectations of the care a companion animal would need.
Possibly the animal is not the running partner, hunting aid, or guard dog the
owner assumed it would be when purchasing it. Perhaps the pet owner has
lost interest in keeping the animal or it sheds more hair and brings more dirt
into the house than expected. A new child, boyfriend, or girlfriend could be
allergic to the species or have an aversion to the animal.

From the perspective of the veterinarian, justifying euthanasia requests
for these cases is difficult because the rationale neglects the value of the animal's life in favor of human convenience. A baby's arrival, a divorce, or a

death in the family could render an animal an inconvenience. In one extreme case, clients requested euthanasia of their black dog because they had recently purchased a white couch and matching carpet. The client argued, "I just can't keep cleaning up after him, and I wouldn't mind it so much if his hair weren't black. It just really shows up against the white couch." Euthanizing healthy animals for the convenience of the owner is considered the least legitimate rationale for euthanasia. Clinton Sanders's research on veterinary euthanasia confirms my findings: "Clients who employed this type of rationale typically were judged to be morally suspect. They were perceived as defining the animal as a piece of property rather than as a sentient being with feelings and interests."[6]

Disagreements over Quality of Life

Veterinarians may disagree with a client's decision to euthanize when they believe the decision is based on an inaccurate assessment of an animal's quality of life.[7] Pet owners may request euthanasia for animals with minor health concerns because, for example, they mistakenly believe the animal is suffering. When the removal of an eye or amputation of a limb is necessary, clients often conclude that euthanasia is in the best interest of the animal. For the veterinarian, this is a mistaken belief due to anthropomorphic bias: "If you would think of amputating one of your legs or having one of your eyes removed, you would think that would be very traumatic, and you might be really depressed about it, but pets don't have that same kind of idea that everybody is looking at them or thinking of them differently, and they just sort of get on with life and do very well." Provided that the animal has few other medical problems, the veterinarian may refuse to euthanize, believing that animals typically have a pretty good quality of life despite missing a limb or an eye.

Veterinarians may not want to euthanize animals with a terminal illness because they believe the animal can live comfortably for some time with the disease before the symptoms become problematic. While a client may request euthanasia for a pet because "it would just be too traumatic to *watch* her get sick or be in pain," to the veterinarian euthanasia can seem inappropriate if the terminal illness has not progressed to a point where the animal's quality of life is poor. As Dr. Browning suggested, most participants try to find a balance between euthanizing a bit too early or slightly too late:

> You feel so good about it [euthanasia] when they are suffering and you are glad that you can end their suffering, but you kind of feel like a killer when they look too good. You don't want to euthanize

an animal right away when you hear the word *cancer* because that animal may have several great months ahead. I like to call the perfect timing, where we euthanize terminal animals, "euthanizing on the cusp," where they haven't started to feel bad just yet but you know it is coming soon, which is really what you want and that is what I want to do with my pets.

Naturally, the definition of too early or too late varies from veterinarian to veterinarian. However, when I asked participants to choose if they would rather err on the side of early or late, most thought it better an animal have a slightly shorter, more comfortable life than a longer one that involves suffering.

Disagreement can also occur when a veterinarian believes an animal has a poor quality of life but the owner believes it is good or at least acceptable. Consider the case of anorexic Molly the shar-pei, a breed of dog known for its distinctive wrinkles. The owners had been syringe feeding her for two and a half weeks. Molly's chart revealed that she had been to the hospital over two dozen times in the last year and recently had surgery to remove a tumor. The oncology department strongly suspected lung cancer, but the tests were inconclusive. Dr. Buford believed that the animal's condition was severe enough to justify euthanasia, but the owners had unrealistic expectations regarding her condition and recovery. The following is an excerpt from my field notes taken while following the case:

> We come out to meet the clients and find a very emaciated brown shar-pei whose ribs and spine are quite pronounced. . . . Because her body is so small but her head remains the same size, it makes the dog look like some rendition of an alien from a science fiction film. She has been too weak to walk on her own for several weeks, so we wheel her back to the exam room, and as we do, other people in the waiting room offer sad looks. Some just stare, and a few even gasp. Dr. B. turns to me and says, "I am so mad at them right now. The owners obviously care for their animal, but they are not being realistic at all. These people are nice but clueless about the condition of this animal. She lost fourteen pounds in two months!"

Cases such as this create considerable buzz among staff members. Staff members in this case expressed strong emotions, including sadness, sympathy (for both the dog and the owners), and anger. From listening to conversations, it became clear to me that many staff believed the owners were being unrealistic in their assessment of the dog's quality of life and, as a result, were making poor decisions that negatively affected the animal's welfare. Several doctors and staff walked by the dog and said, "I am so sorry, girl," or "It is sad, but sometimes they just love their animals so much that they can't see the suffering," or "Sorry, girl. They love you, but they just don't know how to say good-bye." For others, the owner's refusal to euthanize was an act of cruelty. One resident said angrily, "How can you look at this dog and not be able to tell how sick she is?" A nurse who had recently come on shift walked by the dog and, mistakenly believing that it was a case of severe neglect, said, "Wow! Is this a law enforcement case?" The veterinarian sarcastically clarified: "Nope, just cancer and denial."

If the veterinarian believes the patient to be suffering, life-preserving measures (except for pain management) are usually not in the best interests of the animal. In fact, in many of these cases the animals are in such poor condition that they often die before further curative treatment can be administered. If owners see only a minor problem and are unrealistically focused on fixing that, they are caught off guard by a grim prognosis and have difficulty accepting it. Consider the case of a fourteen-year-old, medium-sized, mixed-breed dog who suffered serious injuries when he was hit by a car. The client insisted on doing everything possible to save the animal, but Dr. Logan wanted to euthanize because he believed further treatment would only prolong suffering:

> This case was horrible—truly awful. . . . [The dog] had pulmonary contusions so [it was] bleeding into the lungs, a spinal fracture such that the spine was damaged and there was no motor function in the back legs, and there were four pelvic fractures! Even if he were ever able to use his back legs again, he would need four surgeries to fix the pelvic fractures because both sides were fractured in two areas that were weight bearing and had to be fixed. . . . I was very, very clear with her that not only was the prognosis very poor in general for him to survive but it was extremely poor for him to ever walk again, and he would have to endure multiple surgeries that were very painful. . . . I don't think he is ever going to have a good quality of life again. . . . On all fronts I felt like euthanasia was the right thing to do. She would bankrupt herself, honestly, for a dog that was not going to get better.

In these situations the veterinarian may try to convince clients that it is time to euthanize their animal because they believe that the owner's assessment of the chances for the animal's recovery and quality of life is flawed.

Dying Naturally

Disagreements between clients and veterinarians can be related to the owners not accurately evaluating quality of life, but they can also be related to differences in weighing the value of quantity of life versus quality of life. Veterinarians believe some pet owners prioritize the duration of an animal's life over the animal's quality of life. Many owners are willing to make significant personal and financial sacrifices to have as much time with their companion animal as possible despite its ill health. Other times, clients are ethically opposed to euthanasia and refuse to consider it under any circumstances.

Veterinarians consider the option of euthanasia to end suffering to be a positive aspect of practicing veterinary medicine. They often report a sense of relief when euthanizing an animal with a condition in which suffering is inevitable or pain and distress are already apparent. Thus it can be particularly stressful for the veterinarian when faced with an owner who is ethically opposed to euthanasia. Some owners believe that taking their companion animal home to die naturally would be less stressful than euthanasia, but veterinarians often disagree with such conclusions. Dr. Thomas argued that dying naturally may not be the peaceful experience that clients hope for: "People just have this image that dogs tend to just die peacefully in their sleep. I don't know if humans do that or not, but animals definitely don't do that. . . . Every time I have seen an animal die it looks horrible. Maybe their death is sudden, but what leads up to death is usually pretty horrible."

Managing Disagreement

Pet owners consult the veterinarian as a medical expert with knowledge of animal injury and disease; however, the animal patient is legally their property, and they have the right to decide its fate. When clients make requests that challenge veterinarians' sense of responsibility to their animal patients, it can be difficult for them to comply. Rather than consenting to the client's request, veterinarians use various strategies to negotiate an alternative course of action for their patient. This section describes the approaches veterinarians use to resolve the sorts of disagreements outlined previously.

Providing Knowledge

Educating owners about, for example, proper nutrition and dental hygiene is a daily occurrence for many veterinarians. Sometimes clients make life-and-death decisions based on a misunderstanding, so veterinarians provide knowledge to correct factual errors. In some situations the veterinarian believes that the client mistakenly exaggerates the seriousness of the animal's condition. For example, even if an elderly animal displays no obvious symptoms of pain, owners commonly believe that their older animals are suffering simply because of their age.

Disagreements between client and veterinarian arising from an owner's false impression are often easily dispatched. Consider the owner who wants to euthanize her dog who has just been diagnosed with cardiac arrhythmia because she mistakenly believes the animal might suffer a painful death:

> I told that woman, "You know, the nice thing about sudden death is it is quick. Their heart begins beating irregularly, and the brain doesn't get enough oxygen, and they just faint. If I had to choose, I think that is a pretty nice, reasonable way to go. I just want to assure you that your dog is going to feel fine, and then maybe one day he might just die suddenly, but that is going to be a sudden and painless death, so I think it really would be the right thing to give him whatever good time he has until then." When people [get past] the fear that the situation provokes in them, they are usually okay, but you have to just educate them about certain medical things they may not understand.

Clients may initially consider euthanasia because they overestimate the necessary effort to care for their animal. In these cases, education may include teaching owners techniques for procedures they anticipate will be especially difficult, such as giving daily insulin shots to their diabetic dog or coaching them on how to restrain their cat in order to give daily pills.

Providing knowledge can also help veterinarians convince clients that euthanasia is in the best interest of their animal. Veterinarians often have to educate owners regarding the strong commitment required to care for animals that have lost autonomic function or require chronic management.[8] Once the veterinarian explains that they will have to provide assistance with the most basic functions of life, such as eating and elimination, owners are less resistant to the idea of euthanasia. For example, when a client brought his middle-aged springer spaniel to the hospital with a complaint of lethargy and heavy breathing, he had no idea of the severity of his dog's condition. An examination determined that the dog likely had a condition known as immune mediated hemolytic anemia (IMHA), a disease that causes rapid deterioration and is associated with a high mortality rate.

Initially, the owner adamantly refused to consider euthanasia. The veterinarian then described the condition. Patients with IMHA are often unstable and need at least one blood transfusion as well as high doses of a corticosteroid that can have serious side effects. Patients often do not make it through the treatment and an especially unlucky patient may require weeks of intensive hospitalization before responding. After sitting with the owner for nearly an hour, answering his questions and educating him on the details of the disease, the odds of a successful treatment, and expectations of a rapidly worsening condition, the client came to share the veterinarian's conclusion that euthanasia was in the best interest of the animal.

Providing Alternatives to Euthanasia

Disagreements over whether to euthanize an animal can be solved by the veterinarian providing an appealing alternative. When clients request euthanasia of healthy, well-behaved patients, veterinarians may offer to take over ownership of the animal or place the animal in a local shelter. Requests for the euthanasia of animals with minor health problems can be more complicated to resolve because they require resources to restore them to health before they can be adopted. Consider the case of a three-year-old black-and-white, otherwise-healthy rabbit with a large skin laceration:

> He was a drop-off, so I called the guy up to ask more questions about why he wanted this perfectly healthy, adorable, hopping-around-the-room bunny with a scratch to be euthanized. . . . I could hear in the background these kids screaming, and he says, "Well, actually, I have kids, and we have a lot of rabbits, and we are just not able to invest that much." So I said, "Well this is obviously treatable, and I am not comfortable euthanizing, . . . but there is a rescue organization for bunnies in Santa Barbara, and we will be willing to fix the wound up." The owner was happy to surrender him. . . . It is not always easy to confront clients like that, but sometimes you have to have the courage to just give them other options.

Thus, in certain cases, the veterinarian will treat the animal free of charge if the owners sign over custody to a local animal shelter.

Animal shelters have limited resources to treat sick animals and often have to euthanize those with any illness, therefore the option to give the animal to a shelter applies only to young animals with a fair to good prognosis. Animals that have a less favorable status concurrent with other factors such as older age or lengthy recovery time are often the most difficult to find alternatives to euthanasia. Surrendering these animals to a shelter is generally not a better solution, as the shelter would most likely decide to euthanize them anyway. In very rare cases animal shelters or rescue organizations may have special funds set aside to cover medical expenses, but these funds are generally quite limited. Veterinarians can sometimes convince rescue organizations that certain candidates (who may be less than ideal) are worthy of their limited resources.

Many veterinarians were not comfortable euthanizing animals for assorted behavioral reasons until alternative solutions were at least attempted. Owners with animals that misbehaved by digging holes, barking, or destructively chewing things were encouraged to give the animal more attention or exercise before they considered euthanasia. Owners were also encouraged to explore medical treatment for troublesome behaviors. While veterinarians had few alternatives for seriously aggressive animals, they often suggested owners try medications such as Prozac for minor aggression. Before euthanizing cats for sharpening their claws on furniture, veterinarians encouraged clients to put plastic covers on cat's nails, limiting their ability to damage furniture. Some even recommended having the cat declawed, a procedure many veterinarians find objectionable but superior to euthanasia.

When allergies to the animal were the rationale for euthanasia, veterinarians suggested a variety of alternatives. Clients were encouraged to consider taking allergy medication in combination with keeping animals out of bedrooms. Frequent vacuuming and grooming were also suggested to help reduce hair and dander in the home. A couple of veterinarians even suggested owners go so far as remove all of the carpeting in the home to avoid euthanizing the animal. If clients attempted alternative measures but the troublesome conditions were not eliminated, veterinarians would more readily agree to euthanize. Thus, a veterinarian might come to agreement with an owner's wish for euthanasia after the owner made good-faith efforts to find an alternative.

Identifying Support Networks

Support networks may provide financial aid when lack of resources is the source of dispute between the veterinarian and the client. For example, although veterinarians often hate talking with clients about money, they recognize it is an important part of providing health care to animals.[9] Helping clients identify people in their social network who may be willing to lend funds can prevent financially based euthanasia. Dr. Smith explained:

> Initially, a lot of people say they don't have money, like seriously, 50 percent of the time people say they don't have the money. Then

you say, "Well, a lot of people don't have $2,000 available in their checking account, but . . . can you borrow money from friends or"— if they are young—"maybe your parents?" If they really want to treat, they will be calling their friends, grandparents, aunts, and uncles, and . . . they will get a cosigner for a loan, because we have to get the deposit or they have to get approved for CareCredit [a health care credit card], or they surrender their pet.

Some participants even suggested people call their church to ask for assistance or hold a fund-raiser for their animal.

When owners are having a difficult time saying good-bye to their dying companions, veterinarians also encouraged them to consult others in their support networks in the hopes that their friends would advise euthanasia: "Is there someone else you could call to talk this through?" Veterinarians believed some owners lived with an animal's progressively debilitating condition for so long that they became acclimated and could not see how the animal's quality of life had deteriorated. Veterinarians encouraged owners to phone family members and trusted friends and ask them to come to the hospital for comfort and support: "Is there someone who knows Buster who might want to come and visit him in the hospital?" The veterinarian's hope was that the friend would see the animal's dramatically declined condition and help the owner choose euthanasia, ending the disagreement.

Exploring Quality-of-Life Meanings

Exploring clients' perspectives on their animal's condition can be an important tool in helping resolve disputes. Recognizing that quality of life is subjective, the veterinarian will first establish the owner's goals for quality of life. To determine why a client is requesting or refusing euthanasia, veterinarians will ask open-ended questions to uncover details shaping the client's decision: What do you consider to be a good quality of life for Clyde? What are your concerns for him? Tell me what you understand about Clyde's disease. What do you want for him and your family? What would a quality death look like? How will you say good-bye? When you look back on Chester's death six months from now what will be important to you? What is the worst thing that could happen regarding his death?

Veterinarians may encourage owners to think about what animals like or prefer doing, what their interests are, and what opportunities they have to fulfill these interests.[10] Because many veterinarians consider these subjective aspects of an animal's life to be important factors in determining quality of life, they must rely, at least in part, on owners' assessment of their animal's feelings and general personality. Of course, the veterinarian's underlying assumption is that owners have the ability to accurately report their animals' feelings.

The next step for the veterinarian is to help make the process feel more objective for owners by establishing mutually agreed on categories for monitoring the pet's condition. For example, the veterinarian will ask owners to identify activities the animal particularly enjoys and have them monitor and record the animal's interest in these activities:

> Make a list of what he likes to do. What are the things that made life good? Can she go and play with the dogs in the park? Does she run? Does she play in the water or sit on her favorite windowsill? Whatever it is that your animal likes to do, are they doing that? Because if they are, then maybe they should keep going, but if they're not, I think that is another way of giving them a stopping point. You need to week by week decide on things that he needs to start doing or when enough is going to be enough.

The veterinarian may also ask the owner to monitor medical signs of illness such as loss of appetite, reduced activity, or difficulty breathing. Requesting the client to report updates in the animal's health status also allows the veterinarian the opportunity to reiterate the desired outcome.

Helping owners define quality of life can be an excellent way for veterinarians and clients to reach a compromise. For example, in the following case, the owners set their goals for quality of life for their dog far more broadly than many veterinarians in the hospital would have preferred:

> Some people draw the line at, you know, they don't want to put their animals through chemo or radiation or some of the surgical procedures. Others go further. One dog here had a tumor that was occluding urine flow through its bladder, so we put in a kind of a weird port where the owner had to drain the urine out of the bag several times a day, every day. Some people would think that's [going] way too far. . . . Even some vets would say, "Well, that's going too far. The dog can't even pee; that's [going] too far." . . . So the line is drawn differently for everyone.

Dr. Stevens was careful to set limits for owners resistant to euthanasia: "I believe that euthanasia is not a wrong choice right now for Clyde, but if you want this intervention, we need to talk about monitoring his quality of life and setting some limits." For hospitalized animals, the veterinarian will work with the owner to establish an objective point to stop treatment, as this veterinarian explained to a client whose animal had severe respiratory problems: "There is a chance that your dog will need to go on a ventilator. You have to decide when that time comes if you want to go that far."

By helping clients establish goals for quality of life that are easily monitored, the veterinarian is often able to alleviate the client's anxieties and come up with a compromise that honors both of their preferences. Dr. Miller described her strategies for compromise in situations in which she believes owners are choosing euthanasia too soon:

> If you have a cancer that you find early, and it is at a stage where the animal is not symptomatic, but you know it will be fatal, sometimes they want to euthanize right away, and I usually don't like them to do it right away, so I want to talk about it a bit more. If they say, "I don't want him to suffer," I try to make a pact with them: "I think Fluffy is feeling pretty good right now, and I know that it concerns you that Fluffy is going to get sick, but why don't we set up a few quality-of-life things that you are not willing to live with, and the day she stops whatever those things are, like eating or playing ball, you will bring her in, and we will put her to sleep. Right now, I think she is feeling okay, so let's give her a little bit of time, and the minute she looks like she is not feeling well, then bring her in, and absolutely we won't let her suffer." It makes them feel safe by outlining some parameters to shape quality of life. So you can circumvent them choosing euthanasia that early by talking to them about quality of life.

Veterinarians negotiate with clients to reach a reasonable compromise over when quality of life indicates it is time for euthanasia.

Building Rapport

Veterinarians and owners come to mutually agreed on decisions much more easily when they have good rapport, established during wellness appointments. However, that rapport is most vulnerable during life-and-death decision making.[11] A veterinarian who makes his or her disagreement known to a client can offend or embarrass the client, seriously threatening the rapport. As Dr. Madfis explained:

It is a matter of tact. You don't want to confront them and call them unethical or terrible people. I think you can approach it so you don't make them feel guilty, because I wanted him to be in compliance with what I was asking for . . . even though I thought, "What the fuck? Why are you euthanizing this perfectly healthy animal?" The way to approach it with tact is to say, "Well, I don't know if you are aware, but there are actually some options to consider, like rehabilitating behavior issues." You just present your argument with tact and not like you are passing judgment. It is a really easy thing to do, and people respond really well to that.

Because they are challenging the owner's request, veterinarians recognize that their argument must be delicately phrased to not be interpreted as offensive and that they will more often be successful if their argument is interpreted as sympathetic rather than condemnatory.

Establishing rapport influences client satisfaction with the veterinarian and adherence to the veterinarian's recommendations.[12] In the case of a five-year-old calico cat named Hannah, an intern believed that a resident's disregard for rapport with the owner was to blame for the owner giving up, stopping treatment, and choosing euthanasia:

[This resident] is one of those vets that will just basically . . . lose credibility with the owners. . . . The worst thing about this case was the cat was getting better, but the resident pushed the client so far that he just refused [to authorize further treatment]—that was it. . . . And then one day the cat was eating and was looking better, and the guy said, "I'm done. I want to euthanize.". . . Now all of the sudden all that stuff that the guy would have completely gone for three days ago [is] out of the question because he doesn't trust you.

From this experience, the intern learned that an important part of rapport with owners is making them a key part of decision making at every stage of treatment and not pushing owners into euthanasia decisions or coercing them to treat:

You have to have the owner involved in making decisions. It doesn't mean you don't recommend the best for the patient, but you still work *with* them, and they're much more understanding when it doesn't work. I think when you push them, you get them to a point where

they're not ready to spend all this money, and you basically made
them spend $4,000, and what you're going to end up with is the same
thing you would have ended up with if they spent $1,000—a dead
animal—except now they're going to be really pissed off.

The intern considered the resident's lack of rapport unethical and, perhaps
more importantly, ineffective.

In emergency hospitals, veterinarians often have no prior relationship
with owners, thus it is essential to quickly establish rapport.[13] Veterinarians
establish rapport by using compliments and expressing empathy: "How
are you doing? I know his illness has been difficult for you, and I can see
that you are taking excellent care of Mr. Wiggles." They might even share
personal stories of their own experiences with companion animals when
appropriate.

When clients consider euthanasia because they cannot afford veterinary
services, they may feel angry, embarrassed, or guilty. The veterinarian carefully ensures rapport is preserved by saying, "Of course, no one would expect
you to choose the needs of your animal over the needs of your children, but
I believe Goliath's condition should be treated, and if the shelter is willing to
do it, I think we should go that route." Rapport is preserved by reassuring
owners that a lack of funds is not a reflection on their relationship with their
animal and does not make them a bad pet owner. The same technique also
applies when the veterinarian would prefer that an owner choose euthanasia:
"I can see that you love Tiger, and I can only imagine how much it hurts to
see him like this. He is in a lot of pain right now and is having trouble breathing, and we need to think about what is best for him." The veterinarian pre-
serves rapport by acknowledging the owners' feelings while also encouraging
them to reconsider their decision.

Participants strongly believed that owners were much less likely to resist
the veterinarian's suggestion if they feel the veterinarian is sympathetic to
their situation: "These people are clearly not ready to euthanize, so if I start
right off the bat pushing euthanasia, I am going to lose their trust. They are
just going to think, 'Oh, this doctor doesn't get it.' Then they think they
just have to be defensive and they won't listen at all, and you have no hope
to change their minds." Research on end-of-life communication supports
participants' conclusions regarding the connection between end-of-life conversations, clinical outcomes, and client satisfaction.[14] As this veterinarian
suggested, empathy can be instrumental: "You can't just state your case and
they will go along with it. You need to empathize with them and see where
they are coming from and what factors are important to them. Really know

what they are feeling. When you put yourself in their shoes, it is not always comfortable, but it is helpful in reaching a compromise."

The importance of communication skills in veterinary medicine is an emerging topic.[15] Veterinary clinician Myrna Milani has a column in the *Canadian Veterinary Journal* in which she discusses "the art of private veterinary practice" and often examines the issue of improving client compliance with the veterinarian, as well as veterinarian-client communication.[16] When veterinary articles talk about veterinary communication they typically reflect the experiences of my study's participants. Some articles focus on veterinarians' ability to engage and empathize with clients,[17] while others focus more on their ability to educate and enlist the client's compliance.[18] Recognizing the importance of good rapport and communication skills, many veterinary experts argue that veterinary education should include the teaching of communication.[19]

Confrontation

If the owner has not responded to other strategies and a difference of opinion continues, a veterinarian may intensify expressions of disagreement. Sometimes, confrontation may mean simply ignoring the client's subtle hints:

> Sometimes it becomes obvious [to me] that [clients] were searching for a reason to euthanize, and it can be really frustrating. Like, one animal came in with pretty severe what seemed to be a flea allergy, dermatitis, and [she was] just an older dog. . . . So the husband would say things like "Oh, you think she's in really bad shape?" And I would say, "I think we could treat this." It's almost like a hot potato kind of thing. Who's going to say it? Even though we both know what's going on here. Who is going to call it out? They say things like "Don't you think he looks bad? Do you think he's in pain? Do you think his quality of life is really poor? He's really old." You answer, "I think he still looks pretty good for his age, and no, I don't think he is in pain." I think, "Oh, great. They are searching for justification." And I didn't really want to give it, so I ignore[d] their hints.

Sometimes the veterinarian will strongly advocate for patients by directly challenging the decisions of pet owners as unethical choices:

> Sometimes I will strong-arm the owners, and I will guilt-trip them because my feeling is they are really doing the wrong thing by their

pet. It is kind of nice when you can use their guilt to your advantage to make them treat, because it is so annoying to have to push for treatment for things that should be treated. This is a fixable problem. This is not a reason to kill your pet. It is unethical. You need to find a way to come up with the money. . . . If I feel like they have the financial means but they are being too cheap to do it, I push a little harder.

Ideally, veterinarians want owners to make their own autonomous, informed decisions; however, sometimes the veterinarian believes clients are emotionally overwrought and have lost perspective, rendering them unable to make rational decisions. In one case the family dog had been unable to walk for a year and a half, but the owners did not want to euthanize: "These people were actually expressing this dog's bladder three times a day, and it came to the point where the woman was actually—to help induce the dog to defecate—was pretty much giving the dog a rectal exam." Dr. Thomas confronted the owners, suggesting that the dog was suffering to the extent that she considered it cruel to keep him alive. Two days after this conversation, the owners brought the dog back in for euthanasia:

So, I think, they almost needed that little slap in the face, or on the wrists, like "Hey! Listen, maybe you've been accustomed to this now, but, whoa, what are you doing? Come on. How would you like to have your bladder expressed every day and get a rectal just to defecate?" I think that kind of opened their eyes a bit. I think it's easy for these people to just kind of be so attached and they just get used to or are accustomed to such a horrible way of living, and your normalcy scale is off. They sort of need to be calibrated in a sense.

Most veterinarians do not want to directly confront their clients. Often the first strategy they try is more subtle. For example, Dr. Lawrence knew clients were coming to visit their cat in the intensive care unit. He said, "I am going to leave the BP [blood pressure] cuff on and take the blanket off when they arrive just so they see how bad this situation actually is. I don't want to scare them, but this sucks. Well, maybe if it scares them a little, it will slap some sense into them." Unfortunately, the strategy did not work as Dr. Lawrence had hoped, and he finally reluctantly told his clients that he thought the cat was suffering: "I used very plain words like 'death' and 'starving' and 'suffering.' You have to break out those words sometimes. I try not to because you are almost being nasty with them, but if they need to understand, they need to hear those words." Dr. Lawrence was blunt because he thought his patient was in significant pain and discomfort.

Though veterinarians usually do not feel compelled to use such confrontational words with clients, they often confront them through difficult conversations regarding the reality of death. For example, Dr. Edwards explained how she responds to clients who are ethically opposed to euthanasia: "Generally, I usually just say, 'I am an advocate for the pet.' And then I get a little bit frank, and I will say, 'Death isn't like it is in the movies.' . . . The reality is some animals may simply die in their sleep with no obvious signs of pain or distress, but most will experience a prolonged decline lasting hours, days, or even sometimes weeks, during which organ systems shut down one by one until the animal dies." Veterinarians will explicitly tell owners what to expect when the animal dies in the hope that it will convince them to choose euthanasia. Even if the disagreement is not solved, veterinarians may be relieved that they did the best they could for the patient by expressing their opinion to the client.

Lying and Misrepresenting the Cost of Treatment

Intentionally lying to a client is considered especially unethical behavior among most veterinarians; however, in rare circumstances, veterinarians believe their obligation to be honest with clients could be outweighed by their obligation to protect the interests of the patient.[20] In one such case, a participant lied to a client who was seeking euthanasia for his healthy cat because he was moving to an apartment that did not allow pets. After the client had adamantly refused the veterinarian's offer to place his healthy animal in a local shelter, the veterinarian indicated that he would euthanize the client's animal. Instead, the veterinarian gave the cat to a friend. Although he felt bad for deceiving the owner, he also felt justified in doing so to save the animal's life. However, this behavior is considered highly suspect and could cost a veterinarian his or her license to practice.

Sometimes veterinarians seek to circumvent disagreement with clients by surreptitiously manipulating the cost of treatment.[21] Dr. Jacobs explained how he sometimes exaggerates estimates to try to influence client decisions in his favor, whether to treat or euthanize:

> If you fill out a low estimate knowing very well that the total cost is going to be higher than the estimate, you can get people to admit their pets. And after they've made that investment, yeah, you can

probably get them to keep coming up with money. And at the same time if there is a patient that you think euthanasia would be a better option [for], yeah, you could potentially come up with a giant estimate and force them to make a decision. And I like to think I don't do that. I try to just come up with honest estimates, and I kind of feel like I'm in the wrong when I come up with a low estimate knowing that it's probably going to be higher because I just want to get the patient in the hospital and start treating them.

Although manipulating the expected costs of treatment to sway the client is sometimes tempting to help a patient, it compromises a veterinarian's sense of duty to the owner. Such a strategy comes at a moral cost to the veterinarian, who may feel as though he or she is violating ethical obligations to the owner. However, participants occasionally felt justified in lying or using deception in favor of their judgment as to the best course of action for an animal.

In some cases, sufficient ambiguity in potential medical outcomes allows veterinarians to paint a low-cost, more hopeful picture or a costly, less optimistic picture for the owner without feeling as though they are violating ethical obligations to clients. Indeed, research suggests that it is difficult to give accurate estimates of many chronic, incurable, but not-yet-fatal illnesses.[22] For example, in one study of dogs with congestive heart failure, although a poor prognosis in general, clinicians often gave short estimates of survival time to avoid giving clients unrealistic hope, and such prognoses were the most important factor owners used in making the decision to euthanize.[23] However, the bigger moral conflict for veterinarians is whether it is justifiable to withhold or manipulate information even though that is not, technically speaking, lying to owners.[24] While participants believed occasional deception was justified, most tried to avoid it. They found deception especially distasteful if the veterinarian's motives were for profit rather than the best interest of a patient.

Bargaining for Treatment

When owners do not have enough money to treat their animal, they may reluctantly choose euthanasia. To avoid euthanizing animals in this situation, the veterinarian may bargain with the owner for less expensive treatment plans. For a broken bone, for example, the most expensive option is usually orthopedic surgery and less expensive options might include a splint or cast. The best fracture-repair options vary case by case and many factors go into deciding the best course of action, such as the severity of the fracture, the patient's age, and the type of trauma that caused the break. To avoid euthanizing animals with broken bones, the veterinarian might offer the less expensive but obviously less ideal treatment. For example, the veterinarian may offer limb-removal surgery or another last resort solution:

> I had a cat that got hit by a car, with a fractured pelvis, that the owners couldn't afford surgery [for], but it was urinating and defecating fine, which is the main concern when their pelvic canal is crushed. . . . It wasn't a break that could be bandaged, because it is the pelvis, and so it came down to "What else can we do?" We euthanize the animal or think of another plan, so I had them put their cat in a box for six to eight weeks, with pain meds, and it will heal. It will heal incorrectly, but they will still have a functional cat—hopefully. Obviously, you warn them that it may not [be functional] and [that] we may end up euthanizing, but we gave it our best shot given the financial situation.

Although the least optimal plan can be a frustrating compromise for veterinarians, sometimes it is considered a better alternative to euthanasia.

Choosing the least expensive plan is inherently risky for the patient. Recognizing that treatment options generally fall along a continuum with the most effective (often the most expensive) at one end and the least effective (often the least expensive) at the other, the most medically ideal treatment plans are often jokingly described as Cadillac plans:

> I will offer the Cadillac treatment, and if they decline that, I will say, "Let me revise the estimate, and we will be more conservative, and it is not going to be ideal, but let's see what we can do." And I will keep squeezing the estimate down. I will bargain my way down, and if there is a decent chance they [the patient] will make it and that is the only thing the owner can afford, that is always a better option than just euthanasia. . . . There are ways that you can cut corners, and you don't want to, but it depends on how sick the animal is. So can you get them through the night with something really minimal? . . . With many money cases, you are hoping for a little bit of luck to intervene on your side. . . . Now if [the pet] is really sick or they're [not responding], I would never negotiate if I thought the pet would go home and not do well. Is it ideal? No, but you give 'em some pain meds and hope.

Experienced veterinarians rely heavily on their clinical knowledge to inform them on which animals are likely to survive or do well with a compromised, less ideal treatment plan. If there is a fair chance that the animal can heal and have a good quality of life, veterinarians are willing to compromise quality of care and gamble on the chance that the treatment will be successful.

A veterinarian must take an owner's financial limitations into account when trying to merely determine what might be wrong with the animal. Owners may set particularly narrow limits regarding how much they are willing to spend on their animal's care: "I have $200. What can you do to fix my animal that doesn't cost more than that?" These financial limitations can be so narrow that the veterinarian is unable to medically determine a diagnosis. For example, without diagnostic tools such as a radiograph or biopsy, a veterinarian cannot know whether a palpated mass is a benign or malignant tumor.

For an animal that likely has a condition the owners could not afford to treat anyway, obtaining an exact diagnosis is futile. In other cases there is always hope that a few simple tests could prove the patient has an easily treatable condition. Thus, the veterinarian may skillfully select diagnostic tests to determine whether a condition is treatable or more serious. In other words, with limited funds the veterinarian may not be able to provide an exact diagnosis but could confirm a condition serious enough that euthanasia is acceptable.

Bargaining for treatment did sometimes mean that the veterinarian provided treatment without charging clients. For example, diagnostic tests were done under the table and animals were given restorative fluids or pain medication without charging the owners. Sometimes this was done with colleague and hospital administration approval, but often it was not sanctioned. Hiding tests and treatments from administrators in teaching hospitals is especially risky for interns or residents, whose cases are reviewed by supervisors who might question missing charges or unbilled tests. Veterinarians who provide covert services might avoid disagreements with owners who would otherwise choose euthanasia, but they risk reprimand and damaged relationships with colleagues.

When veterinarians negotiate with owners, it is typically over the number and kinds of services, not the cost of individual services. Although private practice veterinarians had more flexibility than those in large hospitals, they rarely negotiated with owners by offering to lower the price of services. However, to avoid euthanizing animals because of financial costs, they were known to call around to other practices or hospitals to see if their rates were less expensive.

Refusing the Owner's Request

After trying several strategies, sometimes the only plan left is to oppose the client's request and insist on another course of action. Veterinarians sometimes refused an owner's request for euthanasia because they believed the request reflected a disregard for the animal: "There was no way I was going to let that man think that he could just throw his cat out like it was trash. He sure got a piece of my mind on that issue." Several veterinarians refused owners' requests for euthanasia for healthy, easily adoptable animals, resulting in either the owner leaving the hospital with their animal (usually angry and upset) or the animal being released to the care of a local shelter. Even though the veterinarians knew the shelter would likely euthanize the animal, they were comforted by the thought of having given the animal a chance to be adopted, no matter how small the likelihood.

While nearly all veterinarians had refused to euthanize at least one animal in their career, less than a handful had ever refused to stop treating animals, even if they strongly believed that it was better for the animal's welfare to be euthanized. Most veterinarians carried out life-saving treatment regardless of how imprudent it seemed to them or how bleak the outcome appeared. When it came to keeping animals alive, despite their own apprehension, most veterinarians felt obligated to at least oversee their pain management. In fact, several veterinarians had refused to release an animal from the hospital because they believed that the animal would suffer without medical intervention.

Such difficult disagreements are often unable to be resolved because clients deny the deterioration in their animal's condition or refuse to accept that the animal is dying. Dr. Stone had clients who asked to take a nine-year-old German shepherd with multisystem organ failure home: "I wouldn't let that dog leave. I looked at them and said, 'Listen, if this was a human being, there would be no negotiation of her leaving the ER.' There was not going to be any negotiation on that pet leaving this hospital." If owners insist on taking their animals from the hospital the veterinarian will have the owner sign an AMA form, meaning that the owner is taking the animal home "against medical advice" of the veterinarian. In extreme cases, a veterinarian might report an owner to the local authority assigned to deal with animal cruelty.

Most often, however, negotiations do not take such a confrontational turn. The veterinarian will make an initial suggestion of euthanasia to the owner, who rejects the offer and makes a counter-request for continued treatment or longer palliative care. Later, after additional tests and monitoring indicate that the animal's condition is worse, the veterinarian will make another attempt to carefully argue for euthanasia. Regardless of how improbable it seems for the animal to recover, some clients continue to disagree with the veterinarian, and the negotiation continues at a later date. This process may be repeated several times, lasting days, weeks, or even months, depending on the disease process, until either a decision is reached to euthanize the animal or the animal dies on its own.

Abiding by the Owner's Wishes

Bargaining with owners to euthanize a sick animal or avoid euthanizing a treatable one required more confrontation than some veterinarians were comfortable initiating. When clients walk in requesting euthanasia for animals, for example, veterinarians have to find a balance between getting enough information to be comfortable doing the euthanasia and feeling as though they are interrogating emotionally distraught owners. Some participants were so uncomfortable with interrogating distraught pet owners that they did as clients requested without much questioning. Others ignored their own discomfort and abided by owners' requests for practical reasons: "If I am pretty sure this animal is going to get euthanized in the shelter anyway, I might as well get some money for the hospital by doing the euthanasia here." At times, participants went along with owners' requests to preserve their relationship with the client.

Many veterinarians reluctantly abide by an owner's wishes when all other pragmatic or reasonable options for the patient have been exhausted. Dr. Black did not want to euthanize her feline patient in chronic renal failure who required fluid injections every day, for example, but she was realistic that her patient had few other options: "What are the viable options for this cat? Is it adoptable? No, it is not. If this owner doesn't want it and isn't going to take good care of it, it is reasonable to elect euthanasia." She further defended her choice:

> Say if you have a case with, say, a seventeen-year-old dog who has some health problems but is getting along okay, but . . . the owners are moving and it is some kind of bullshit convenience thing. What are you going to do with a seventeen-year-old dog? Are you going to put it in a shelter? Are you going to take it away from everything it has known? Is that a kind thing to do? It is actually not. It is not fair to really old pets to put them through that kind of a change and that kind of stress, not to mention that they won't be adopted. That means they will spend the rest of their lives in a cage, and it sucks that the owners are abandoning them at that age for some reason that doesn't have to do with a health concern, but at the same time, that is their right, and realistically there are no good other options for this animal.

Dr. Black colorfully concluded, "You might look at it realistically and think, 'What is the ideal thing for this animal?' The ideal thing is that the owner would not fucking suck, but the owner fucking sucks, so there are no good options, so you do the euthanasia." Veterinarians often reluctantly abide by owners' wishes because they believe there are no better options for the animal.

Though pet owners and veterinarians often reach agreement regarding life-and-death decisions for companion animals, disagreements sometimes occur and must be carefully navigated to avoid damaging the veterinarian-client relationship. For example, clients may become upset with the veterinarian because they feel they have been accused of unethical behavior or they may resent the veterinarian's interference as unwarranted and intrusive. Because heated negotiations are stressful for the veterinarian and can potentially cause anger and lasting resentment in the client, veterinarians patiently and tirelessly work through differences with clients so that an understanding can be reached. Sometimes veterinarians easily dispatch disagreements using only one strategy, but other times they must try several strategies before navigating a disagreement and arriving at a harmonious arrangement.

Although serious disputes are relatively rare, nearly every participant had experienced at least one situation in which an amicable solution to a disagreement could not be reached. An example is a client who wanted to take her cat home because she thought he was well enough to leave the hospital, but the veterinarian disagreed and had her sign against-medical-advice paperwork. The client yelled in the busy lobby that the veterinarian was "trying to kill [her] cat." Many times participants had to curb their anger and frustration and keep the interaction from getting out of hand to avoid a potential lawsuit. Unfortunately, a few veterinarian-client disagreements ended with "You'll hear from my lawyer."

Negotiations can become complicated because of the wide array of attitudes regarding nonhuman animals held by pet owners and veterinarians. For example, the exact circumstance in which euthanasia is considered legitimate can vary dramatically from client to client and veterinarian to veterinarian. When it comes to financing a pet's health care, some pet owners commit to spending relatively little on veterinary care, while others spend thousands of dollars on the most advanced technology available for their companions. Moreover, the veterinarian and client may have drastically different ideas regarding reasonable efforts that pet owners should be morally or ethically obligated to make to provide for their companion animals. To sustain the life of an animal companion some clients are willing to clean up vomit and diarrhea every day during cancer treatments, while others refuse to give their diabetic animal a daily injection. When it comes to euthanizing animals with aggression or other behavioral problems, veterinarians disagree as to how much effort clients should be expected to put forth to change the undesirable or abnormal behavior before agreeing to euthanasia.

Traditionally, the role of the veterinarian is to provide a list of options for the pet owner that vary in cost, quality, and sophistication, leaving nearly every decision regarding their animal patients entirely in the hands of the client. However, as we have seen in this chapter, some members of the profession are beginning to challenge such traditional roles. For example, some veterinarians euthanize healthy, well-behaved animals because their owners no longer want them, while others are morally opposed to this practice. Veterinarians practicing today increasingly refuse to leave treatment decisions entirely up to the owner. No matter how vigorously veterinarians argue their position, however, the animal's owner has the final say regarding the fate of his or her pet. Nevertheless, many veterinarians feel obligated to be advocates for the best interest of animals, just as pediatricians are expected to be advocates for the best interest of children.

2

Creating a Good Death

The Dramaturgy of Veterinary Euthanasia

The care that veterinarians take to create a good euthanasia experience for their animal patients and human clients first became clear to me during a brief but poignant exchange with an intern. Often owners who choose not to be present during euthanasia wish to spend time with the pet's body before it is cremated. While walking down a long corridor carrying the body of a cat we had just euthanized out for the owner to view, the intern said to me, "Hey, does this cat look dead to you?" I responded, "Well I guess so; it is *actually* dead." The intern laughed and said, "I know, but I don't like it if they look *too* dead. It is better if I can make it look like they are just asleep or something." To achieve the desired peaceful appearance, the intern was careful to avoid allowing the animal's head to hang limply from her arms—all for the sake of her human client.

A patient's remains are treated respectfully behind closed doors, but extra care is taken in the presence of clients to ensure the impression that the veterinarian has special consideration for the animal's body. The veterinarian may delicately carry the animal wrapped in a blanket or neatly position the body on a gurney, making sure that a tail or paw does not hang loosely off the side. Acting in much the same way as funeral staff,[1] the veterinarian is careful to talk quietly and walk slowly to preserve the desired impression of gravity. Also, similar to their funeral staff counterparts who are always serious and somber in front of clients, veterinarians may talk loudly and even joke while preparing the body behind closed doors. However, to dismiss either profession's actions in front of clients as insincere is to miss a much more sophisticated reality.

Veterinarians often go out of their way to control the appearance of the dead. To create the most pleasing image, an animal's body may be washed, shaved, or groomed and its eyes are always carefully closed. Any feces or urine excreted after death is wiped clean. The body is sometimes covered with a sheet of disposable absorption padding, towel, or blanket. The veterinarian may even take the time to sew up an open trauma wound or cover disfiguring injuries. This was certainly the case with an iguana named Jax. After radiographs confirmed renal failure, the young male client, his parents, and the veterinarian agreed euthanasia was best. Although the family did not want to be in the room for the procedure, they did wish to be with his body afterward and take it home for burial.

Jax escaped our grasp during the euthanizing process and scrambled off the table. Like many lizards, iguanas can drop, or autotomize, their tails, meaning that their tail breaks off from the body. This ability, of course, comes in most handy when a predator grabs hold of an iguana's tail in the wild, but it can also happen when well-meaning veterinarians try to restrain them. After finally capturing and euthanizing the elusive Jax, Dr. Stevens did not want to present the body of a treasured pet in two pieces to the family. Instead of simply explaining the tail loss as a natural response, he took the time to glue and suture the tail back on the dead lizard. When I asked him why he was doing this, he told me that he did not want the clients to think that their pet suffered a violent death, adding, "Jax just didn't look right or very peaceful without his tail." To finish off his presentation, Dr. Stevens found an appropriately sized cardboard box, lined it with a blue medical pad, and artfully placed the newly restored body of Jax on a makeshift pillow.

Although not an especially typical patient, the story of Jax is not unique. Similar to those in the funeral business, veterinarians diligently work to provide their clients with a specific image of their deceased loved one (although they use much less sophisticated preservation and restoration techniques). Just as funeral directors take pains to create what they call a memory picture for the family,[2] veterinarians believe that euthanasia is an important experience for pet owners because it is the last memory of their pet: "Euthanasia is important to people. That is what they are going to remember as their last few minutes with their animal so it's our responsibility to make sure it goes peacefully." Veterinarians often liken their role in euthanasia to that of a funeral director performing funerals for pet animals. During my time with veterinarians I paid particular attention to how veterinarians frequently go to great lengths to shape euthanasia as a pleasing, personalized, and intimate experience for clients.

From the veterinarian's perspective, the goal of a good client-witnessed euthanasia is a gentle slipping into death, which looks like an animal is quietly and painlessly falling asleep. Ideally, after the necessary paperwork and preparation, the euthanasia solution is delivered smoothly and death comes peacefully in a matter of minutes. Typically within six to twelve seconds after the injection, the pet will take a slightly deep breath, grow weaker, and finally lapse into what looks like a deep sleep (giving rise to the euphemism "put to sleep"). The euthanasia solution primarily consists of a concentrated anesthesia that causes loss of consciousness, numbs pain, and suppresses the cardiovascular and respiratory systems. A few minutes after the injection, the veterinarian listens for the absence of a heartbeat and pronounces the animal dead.

Euthanasia is considered successful when the animal dies peacefully, the veterinarian maintains an appropriate presentation, and the owners are thought to have a good last memory of their pet. No matter how carefully a veterinarian aims for a good death for patients and grieving clients, there are always opportunities for error. Because of the finality of the event, the veterinarian has no opportunity for a second chance and must work diligently to see that the euthanasia performance is as near perfect as possible. Thus, they create routines and procedures designed to tightly control the technical circumstances of euthanasia through the use of backstage preparation, props, tailored spaces, and specific rhetoric. No matter how routine the euthanasia process becomes, however, each procedure must still be brought off, with all the opportunities for error.

Threats to a Good Death and Their Management

In many respects veterinarians and members of their team are actors whose job it is to stage a performance for their audience (the clients and sometimes their friends and family). As with any performance, the concern is likely to be with whether the show comes off or falls flat. Performances are considered successful when the audience perceives the death of the animal to be peaceful and painless and interprets the actions of the veterinarian to be competent, sincere, dignified, and respectful. Every effort is made by the actors to ensure that the euthanasia experience is arranged in a way to create favorable images and impressions. However, much can happen that can contradict the ideal peaceful performance.

Technical Failure

No matter how skilled a veterinarian may be in the technical aspects of euthanasia, the possibility for mishaps remains. The three common routes of administration of euthanasia solution are intravenous (injected into a vein), intraperitoneal (injected into the abdominal cavity), and intracardiac (injected into the heart). When deciding on a route of administration, veterinarians consider their own technical skills, the animal's species, the behavioral nature of the animal, and the degree of injury or illness, as well as how the animal's death may appear to the owner. For example, certain conditions dogs and cats suffer make it difficult or impossible to administer the euthanasia solution by the preferred intravenous route:

> A few months ago I had this ATE [arterial thromboembolism][3] cat who came in agonal [a type of labored respiration][4] because he had thrown a clot. . . . But this cat, his heart had just failed, and there was hardly any blood pressure at all. And that's why he was dying right in front of us, and that's why we couldn't get any kind of a vein. And this cat was in low-output failure. . . . And so I had a very good tech on, and both the tech and I tried on three veins while the owner is standing there.

Intraperitoneal (IP) administration is a method most often used with animals for whom it is too difficult to gain access to a vein (especially exotic animals such as rabbits, hamsters, birds, mice, and reptiles) or dogs and cats who have poor circulation due to disease. This method is technically less efficient (taking as long as half an hour) and less aesthetically pleasing than intravenous injections. Intracardiac (IC) administration is the least used route and the most technically challenging (because it requires the veterinarian to accurately hit a heart chamber). Because it is stressful to conscious animals, this method is typically used on deeply sedated or anesthetized patients and is generally regarded as the most aesthetically displeasing (especially to nonmedical persons).

Although all three routes are considered technically appropriate for a painless death, many veterinarians do not like owners to witness the latter two methods because the death may not appear peaceful or painless:

> I try not to have owners present when we don't really have venous access and have to do IP or IC, which I think is upsetting for owners to see. It is upsetting for me to do, so I would imagine that it would be upsetting for them to see me hold their bird or hamster and stick a twelve-gauge needle into its abdomen or heart. I think that would be perceived as maybe cruel to the owner. Most vets try not to offer witness for exotics. It is harder to make it look peaceful.

Owners are strongly discouraged from witnessing euthanasia of pets for which the necessary method of administration is unable to provide a good, or peaceful, presentation. Several veterinarians refused to allow owners to watch euthanasia unless they are able to use the preferred intravenous route: "I won't do an intracardiac stick in front of an owner. . . . I outright won't euthanize with them present. It kind of looks weird when the animal succumbs to gas anesthesia. I don't want the owners present, because it's like he's dying in a gas chamber, and then you have to stick the heart and we can't always get it on the first try. You know, talk about a shitty euthanasia experience."

Intravenous (IV) administration is the method most often preferred for dogs and cats and is generally considered the most rapid (usually under one minute), predictable, and aesthetically pleasing route for drug administration. However, getting a delicate needle into a squirming patient's vein does not always happen on the first try even for the most experienced veterinarians. When an owner is going to be present for the euthanasia, an indwelling catheter is frequently placed in the pet's vein to ensure that the euthanasia solution is delivered quickly and accurately. Without a catheter in place, an assistant is often needed to help hold the animal and apply pressure to aid in passing the fine needle into the pet's vein. Taking the time to place a catheter is extra work for veterinarians, but many consider this backstage preparation necessary if they are not confident of hitting a vein on the first try.

Veterinarians share a concern for the appearance of a painless, smooth death in an owner-witnessed euthanasia: "They are there to euthanize their animal so the animal doesn't feel any more pain, and the last thing they want to see is you stick it two or three times to hit a vein." Using catheters during euthanasia procedures is often strictly for the benefit of the audience: "I will always have a catheter in if the owner is going to be present. If the owners are not going to be present, I don't think necessarily that the animal needs a catheter, . . . and probably the majority of the time it's going to go fine and it's going to go smooth. But I would just never want it to *not* go smooth in front of an owner." Of course, the veterinarian would rather gain access to a vein on the first try for the sake of the animal, but mistakes are always possible. The catheter ensures that the audience sees the veterinarian as competent and the death of the animal as peaceful.

Restraint is often necessary to euthanize an animal, but the more restraint that has to be used, the more difficult it is for veterinarians to believe the death appeared peaceful to the owner: "I am pretty sure you don't want somebody's last moments with their dog [to be] watching you wrestling their dog down to get an IV in them." One novice veterinarian describes how she learned the importance of minimal restraint while she was a veterinary student:

INTERN: One vet I worked for—I don't know if she just didn't have any common sense or—or what, but she thought it was acceptable to euthanize cats using the jugular vein with the owners present. As the assistant trying to help her, I felt uncomfortable.

AUTHOR: Why was it uncomfortable, specifically?

INTERN: Just, you know, you have to restrain the head; there's a lot more restraint involved, and it's not like the people can be at the head petting the cat. I mean, for the animal it's probably the same either way. I just think for the people it's not as—as, like, aesthetically pleasing to watch their pet being restrained by the head like that.

Most veterinarians take steps to assure that they use as little restraint as possible in the presence of owners. Inserting an indwelling catheter and giving the animal a sedative or tranquilizer are both backstage steps that can be taken to avoid restraining the animal in front of owners: "I would rather sedate a dog than muzzle them or physically restrain them because it just looks like they are less resistant."

Even in the best circumstances mistakes are possible, and nearly every veterinarian could share at least one horror story regarding technical mistakes made during euthanasia. Catheters, for example, can be excellent in helping euthanasia go smoothly, but they are not without failure: "I had a horrible euthanasia where the catheter had come apart, but I didn't know, so I kept on giving injections, and the pet was just sitting there . . . still breathing for a long, long time. . . . So I felt that the wrap on the catheter was wet, so I had to unwrap the entire thing in front of the owners and put it back in. That was embarrassing." Although veterinarians are often distressed or embarrassed by technical mishaps, they generally have techniques to use to avoid drawing the client's attention to the mistake.

Some mistakes are not as easily ignored and, when they occur, make it far more difficult to save the show. For example, a failure to remove monitoring devices can be especially awkward when the animal dies: "Once I forgot to turn off the EKG [electrocardiogram] machine on a dog, and that sucks 'cause then you hear that awful sound when their heart stops. I have forgotten to turn down the rate on the ventilator, which means you are basically ventilating for a dead dog. That is horrible for owners to watch." Dr. Lawrence was equally emphatic:

The last thing you want for critical patients is to leave the pulse ox[imeter (a machine that monitors blood oxygen saturation)] running or to leave the blood pressure or the EKG running and have the alarm go off when you euthanize the pet. I am so careful about that. . . . I'll just turn the machine off so it is not going to get a reading. And another really important thing is to turn off the fluid pump; otherwise, when you clamp off the catheter to give the euthanasia, the fluid pump, after three seconds, is going to beep at you. So right in the middle of the euthanasia the pump's alarm goes off. You've got to make sure nothing is going to interrupt you mechanically and make sure nothing is going to register the death. There's nothing worse than seeing a v-fib [ventricular fibrillation] on an EKG and then the EKG alarm goes off. That's fucking terrible.

Even the most careful and technically skilled veterinarians recognize that mistakes will happen. But, as Dr. Lawrence told me, some mistakes feel so horrible that making them only once ensures that a veterinarian never forgets to prevent them in the future.

Failed Management of the Animal's Biological Reactions

Recognizing that the animal is often the most unpredictable player in the scene, veterinarians manage owners' impressions of the animal before, during, and after the euthanasia. Before the euthanasia process begins, an ideal euthanasia can be disrupted when an animal is thought to look either too sick or too well. If the animal does not seem sick on that day, some owners may second-guess their decision: "It can be heartbreaking when they gobble down treats and are still wagging their tail even though they are really sick." If the animal seems especially affected by an illness, owners may believe they have waited too long and the animal needlessly suffered. Either way, the veterinarian is prepared to ease the client's potential concerns. If the animal looks particularly sick, the veterinarian might say, "Well, at least he won't be suffering anymore," and if the animal looks particularly good, the veterinarian might say, "Well, it is better that his last day was a good day and our last memory of him is a happy one."

During the euthanasia, the veterinarian must continue to monitor and manage the impressions of the owners regarding the animals. If the goal is a gentle slipping into death, much like falling asleep, then the performance is ruined when it appears to the owner as though the animal suffered or when the owner interprets the animal's behavior as unpleasant or disturbing. For example, it can be disturbing to watch a standing animal (especially big dogs) fall to the ground or, worse, fall off a table as they die, so veterinarians usually have the animal lying down while giving the solution.

Popular television images of death may shape owners' expectations of how the death of their pet should appear, adding additional complications for veterinarians when the pet's death contradicts this image: "Hollywood often makes death seem kind of romantic. They don't show you the reality of death, like the person releasing their bowels." After the animal dies, there is complete muscle relaxation, often accompanied by urination and defecation: "And that kind of thing sucks. . . . It's a normal, natural process, but you hate for the whole scene to be seen, like, not as respectful because there is, like, bloody diarrhea all over or vomit. You just wish that would have never happened." Just as funeral directors hide or cover up certain realities of death from family members, veterinarians try to do the same for clients. Thus, if owners are going to hold animals in their laps, veterinarians will often diaper them or wrap them in a towel or blanket to collect urine or feces released after death.

The euthanasia presentation can be tainted or ruined when the animal's physical reactions do not *appear* consistent with a pain-free and peaceful death. Emphasis is placed on "appear" because, although the animal may experience some mild discomfort or a slight burning sensation if the solution goes outside the vein, for the most part veterinarians are confident that the animal is not in pain. However, as Dr. Shelly explained, veterinarians fear the layperson's misinterpretation of some biological reactions:

> You have seen the extensive rigidity and the [*she makes a howling noise*]. I fucking hate that because it sounds so painful, even though I know what it is. [It's] the anesthesia['s] effect on the brain . . . [that] made him wail, but it wasn't pain. . . . And I tried to explain that to the owner afterwards. . . . I wanted them to understand that their dog was not hurting even though it looked weird, and I am sorry that was upsetting. I do want them to know that their pet was *not* really hurting. But when the patient does something weird, that sucks.

When these vocalizations occur veterinarians quickly remind the owner that the pet is no longer conscious and is not experiencing pain.

Even when veterinarians are unsure of what is happening with the animal, they reassure the client that the animal is not experiencing pain. Dr. Brown described the difficult euthanasia of a nine-year-old Irish setter who had a brain tumor:

> I gave the euthanasia solution, and the dog went through all these horrible neurologic signs. . . . It just did all these horrible things that dogs shouldn't do, like its head slid back, it started to howl, all of its legs started to paddle. . . . It was awful. I had to be like, "Yeah, this is

normal for dogs with brain tumors." I actually never had that happen before. [*Laughs.*] I didn't know if it was true or not. . . . You try to stay calm and tell people that it is normal and that they are not feeling anything, and sometimes you are completely making it up.

Even though Dr. Brown had never seen such biological reactions, she believed it was important to reassure the clients that they were typical given the animal's illness. Dr. Thomas had a similar experience: "Once this cat was sort of vomiting foam, and I had never seen that happen before. I told them that with a heart condition these things are normal. I don't know why I said that, 'cause it is *not* normal." Regardless of their own feelings of uncertainty or disgust, participants reassured clients that their animal was not experiencing pain. Yet talking with me behind closed doors, they described the animals' reaction as "shocking" or the most "disturbing thing [they] had ever seen."

After the animal has died, veterinarians must continue to manage the impressions that owners have of their animals. Ideally, the veterinarian listens for a heartbeat and in a few seconds confirms an animal's heart has stopped; however, sometimes the heart may continue beating for a prolonged period. During a seminar on euthanasia I attended at one of the teaching hospitals, a veterinary instructor warned his students to consider this when clients are watching them: "Hearts may continue to beat for a few minutes. . . . You may [want to] wait to check for heartbeat because it may worry the owner if you listen too long. The owners get nervous. Make it seem like you are just taking your time and wait a few minutes before listening for the heart."

Chemicals stored in nerve endings are released, causing occasional muscle twitching in the early postmortem period. Thus, an animal may appear to breathe after the veterinarian has pronounced them dead, as explained by Dr. Turner:

Different patients will act differently. . . . Their heart has stopped, clearly, but they will just have like nerve and muscle reactions after they are gone. Of course, people view that like, 'Oh, my God. He is alive. He is suffering.' I always warn them about it, but even when it happens, it is still weird and embarrassing. It is uncomfortable. [*Laughs nervously.*] It really sucks, . . . but it was just their muscle reflex; . . . that was kind of hard to describe to them. No, your pet is gone. This is just soft muscle spasms, and they just happen.

As with vocalizations, most veterinarians respond by giving medical explanations for these physiological responses: "I usually say that there is nothing to worry about and that they are not in any pain. He is gone, but it is just that oxygen is leaving the muscles. The diaphragm is a muscle, so it can almost look like they take a breath." While most clients are satisfied with the explanation, a few need more convincing that the animal is deceased: "To convince them, I drew up more solution and gave it [to the animal] because otherwise they weren't going to leave. . . . It was clearly not necessary; I mean, I gave a hundred-pound dose to this thirty-pound dog. It was ridiculous. But that was the only way it was going to convince them that their dog was gone."

Given that some potentially problematic biological reactions are not easily altered or hidden from clients, some veterinarians believe that warning owners neutralizes the effect of witnessing them unexpectedly. These veterinarians prepare clients for what to expect as death occurs: the pet's eyes do not close, there may be a last gasping breath that is more of a muscle spasm, there may be vocalization, there may be muscle twitching, the heart may continue beating for a short time after breathing has stopped, and finally bladder and bowel contents will most likely be released. Although some veterinarians give more details than others, the general idea is that the more the veterinarian can do to prepare clients for these possibilities, the less traumatic the experience will be for clients. The key to the successful explanation is to find a careful balance between being too graphic, causing the owner undue anxiety, and not supplying enough information, such that the owner is shocked or confused.

Almost every aspect of owner-witnessed euthanasia is aimed at managing the final impressions of the clients and creating a peaceful death scene. As part of their orientation when they arrive at City Hospital, interns are required to attend a lecture dealing with the performance aspects of euthanasia. Here they learn that even the *rate* at which the animal dies may be altered to create a desirable death scene. Interns are told to consider injecting the euthanasia solution into the stomach to slow the death process: "If you suspect that owners might find the prospect of it happening quickly difficult, you might want to use IP. This is a more 'movie style' death and is what some people expect." As this quotation highlights, interns learn that the *appearance* of a good death in an owner-witnessed euthanasia is as important as any other aspect.

That veterinarians are intensely concerned with eliminating the appearance of suffering does not mean that they are unconcerned with the animals in their care or that they are insincere. On the contrary, most participants consistently demonstrated the utmost concern for their patients and frequently expressed distress when called on to euthanize them. Far from being unsympathetic to the well-being of their patients, they were confident that they were able to make death as quick and painless as possible. It is veterinarians' confidence in their ability to control animal suffering that allows them to shift from seeing the patient as the subject of concern to seeing it as an object within a performance. This cognitive shift allows veterinarians to focus on lessening the appearance of suffering for the sake of nonmedical outsiders without detracting from their ability to make euthanasia as painless as possible for their patients.

Dramaturgy

In his 1959 book *The Presentation of Self in Everyday Life*, sociologist Erving Goffman notes a connection between human behavior in daily life and theatrical performances.[5] He suggests that life is composed of theaters in which we all play out distinct interactions with people in a variety of different settings according to prescribed social roles. In social interaction, just as in theater, "actors" (individuals) perform in front-stage regions for audiences and other times can be in backstage regions outside the view of the audience. The separation of front and back stages is often essential in maintaining the impressions desired for clients. For example, in the funeral business, the deliberate separation helps avoid potential conflict between the bereavement work of the front stage and the "dirty" tasks of the back stage.[6] The work that funeral directors do in the back stage would appear unseemly to family members and ruin the peaceful, resting image of the deceased that funeral staff desire for their audience.

Since Goffman's introduction of his dramaturgical perspective, countless sociologists have demonstrated its applicability in many social and occupational settings, including the work worlds of police officers,[7] topless dancers,[8] overseas tour guides,[9] doctors,[10] nursing home workers,[11] and labor negotiators.[12] Sociologists note how workers in these occupations perform according to certain scripts in front of customers but may act entirely differently out of sight in the back stage. For example, while in the front stage, a flight attendant is expected to be polite even though passengers may be rude and demanding.[13] However, when alone with fellow employees, the same flight attendant may complain about, express anger toward, or make fun of annoying passengers. Similarly, call-center employees hang up the phone and let off steam among colleagues because they are not allowed to display negative emotions while talking with customers.[14]

The Use of the Back Stage

The back stage, hidden from the audience, often masks information that conflicts with the goals of the performance. Goffman reminds us of the need to deliberately separate the front-stage from the backstage region because the preparations for performances, if seen, may contradict or destroy the impressions fostered front stage.[15] If the goal of a euthanasia is to appear peaceful and painless, the audience will have to be kept away from areas where animals might be subject to procedures that are interpreted as painful: "It is pretty easy to inject euthanasia solution if nobody is watching you. If I am putting an animal to sleep without the owners there, I don't put an IV catheter in, but I would if somebody's watching. Poking around to find a vein is not what you want the animal's last memory to be or an owner's memory to be of their animal." Thus, the catheter is placed in the backstage area of the hospital, out of sight of the client.

Outsiders generally have little, if any, relevant information regarding the workings of backstage areas and the performers work hard to restrict outsiders from complete information about these areas. The backstage areas in veterinary hospitals are typically rooms located beyond the lobby and exam rooms. For medical procedures more complicated than taking an animal's temperature, veterinarians ask clients to wait in the examination room while they take outpatients to designated treatment areas (large rooms full of activity with patients on examination tables awaiting the attention of busy nurses and veterinarians transporting medical equipment and supplies). Critical patients are taken back stage to similar workstations in critical care units (CCUs), also known as intensive care units (ICUs). The walls of CCUs are typically lined with stacked steel cages for monitoring critical patients—canine patients on the bottom and feline patients on top. Clients are allowed to visit sick animals in the CCU only during specified visiting hours and approved special occasions.

If the goal is to appear respectful to the patient, the audience will have to be kept away from the areas that might disrupt this image. For example, public access is strictly prohibited to places where bodies are stored or cremated. While some large veterinary hospitals have their own crematorium facilities, most contract with commercial crematoriums. If clients pay for a private cremation and wish to receive their animal's ashes back, the corpse will most likely be placed in a black plastic bag and stored inside a large refrigerated unit until taken to the crematorium. If the corpse is going to group cremation, the body may be stored with others in large buckets or plastic containers.

Veterinary insiders, of course, become accustomed to the reality of backstage procedures. However, several participants recalled their first exposure to the back stage of body storage as particularly upsetting: "It gives you the chills the first time you see that bucket of dead animals or the first time you see an animal's body put into a bag. Now it doesn't really bother me that they are put into bags. I don't think there is a more appropriate means of disposal. I don't find it disrespectful, but it does take some getting used to." A few participants admitted that they have yet to become completely comfortable with the discontinuity between front-stage and backstage handling of bodies:

> Where I did my internship, . . . there was a really high volume and lots of death and euthanasia; we had that awful big bucket of bodies. [*Nervous laughter.*] That was horrible, and I wasn't shocked by it but maybe a little grossed out. Treatment of the bodies and stuff kind of made me sad in a way—that we go through all these efforts to euthanize someone's pet with all this respect and then it is impossible to go through all the body-handling process with that same level of care and respect, especially if you have a pretty high case load. I totally understand [why they store the bodies in that way] for practical reasons, but it is just kind of sad.

That most staff refused to allow their own pets' bodies to be put into plastic bags reinforces the importance of keeping owners out of these areas: "If even the thought of one of our animals being in a plastic trash bag is that disturbing to people who are used to it every day, then imagine how upsetting it would be for owners to see that!"

The Rhetoric of the Back Stage

Safely in the backstage area, veterinarians and staff sometimes employ behavior and language not shown to the front-stage audience. During a euthanasia procedure, for example, veterinarians speak tenderly and with care not to upset grieving clients. Yet behind closed doors, the same busy veterinarian might tersely ask an assistant to help prepare a pet's body for cremation by yelling, "I need a bag and tag in room two." While conversations about death and dying are serious and somber in front of clients, conversations backstage can be lighter and even humorous at times. Therefore, the back stage is not just a space where upsetting tasks are hidden but a space where performers can step out of character without fear of disrupting the performance for the audience.

As discussed in the Introduction and Chapters 4 and 5, dark humor is often a cathartic expression that allows workers to vent about frustrating and emotionally upsetting aspects of their jobs. Because I discuss humor as a coping mechanism in other chapters, I mention it only briefly here. In the words of Dr. Madfis:

> We use that humor to survive. . . . It is not that we don't have respect for the situation, and it is not that we are not sad about the situation. In fact, we joke . . . because we have all these emotions that we have to deal with in some way. That is why we joke. We don't really make light of it in the sense that we don't care and it doesn't matter to us. [We joke] . . . because it matters to us and because we care and because it is awkward and tense and stressful and it is a big responsibility and we take it so personally—that is why we have to come in and [*big sigh*] say, "Whew! Thank God it is over," and it may come out as something funny sometimes. I think any person that routinely deals with death must laugh about it sometimes.

Veterinarians commonly use humor and sarcasm among backstage peers to reduce feelings of anger or frustration that are not considered appropriate to express in the front stage. For example, backstage talk allowed Dr. Hill to let off steam with her colleagues and express anger she felt toward her clients because they requested euthanasia for their cat that would not stop clawing their expensive furniture. Dr. Hill mockingly pretended to respond to her client, "Yeah, no problem. I understand. I had to put down two of my children. They were awful, always throwing tantrums and biting and destroying my furniture." With an exaggerated sigh, she threw her hands in the air and sarcastically concluded, "It was really for the best."

In the front stage an animal's medical condition is exclusively described using technical terminology, but dark or clever euphemisms are sometimes used by workers in the back stage. For example, a serious medical condition known as disseminated intravascular coagulation (DIC) would be called "death is coming" or "dead in the cage," but only in front of fellow veterinary insiders. Animals nearing death are described as brave and strong in front-stage conversations, but in the back stage they may be referred to as "circling the drain," "making the Q sign" (with tongue hanging out), or having "a case of BSBF" (buy small bags of food). Only behind the scenes would dead or dying animals be jokingly referred to as "going PU," or paws up.

Though most staff members considered the back stage a place to let loose from the restraints of their front-stage role, not everyone was completely at ease with some backstage rhetoric. For example, many novice veterinarians initially expressed discomfort with the gallows humor used by senior staff. While newcomers eventually became accustomed to the rhetoric of the back stage, level of participation varied from individual to individual. The pressure novices feel to participate in or at least accept the dark humor of others reminds us that when performers are in the back region they are nonetheless in another performance—that of a loyal team member. Yet in my experience among veterinarians, even the most no-nonsense professionals occasionally joke behind the scenes. Although backstage rhetoric can create divisions among colleagues, it more often strengthened bonds between veterinary coworkers and helped them discuss difficult issues.

Maintaining Strict Boundaries

Backstage rhetoric, preparatory work, and body storage would likely upset or shock nonprofessionals or those emotionally connected to the deceased. Of course, as with any play, performers have much more knowledge than the audience. Audiences are supposed to know only what the performers choose to disclose. Veterinarians, like any good performer, work hard to control their audience's access to insider information, especially when the information, if accidentally revealed, could ruin the entire show:

> There are a lot of things that you try to keep hidden. It is annoying when they [owners] are real high maintenance and they have asked me the same question twenty times and I am acting like . . . I am happy to answer all your questions . . . again for the tenth time. . . . As soon as I get in the back, I fucking roll my eyes and I am like, "These guys are nightmare high-maintenance clients." I vent, but . . . I don't want the owners to hear my comments about their picky personality.

Overhearing the backstage colloquy could have serious consequences, not just for the immediate performance of a euthanasia but also for the hospital as a business. Great care is generally taken to prevent outsiders from hearing backstage talk. As Dr. Miller said, "Of all the things that I would not want people to know, the biggest one is that we ever joke about death or, especially, the death of their pet. I am always really careful. I will get into ICU with the door closed, and they have the door closed in the exam room, and I will still whisper [a joke] to someone else. But I will *never* do it when we are walking in the hallway."

Audience exposure to the back stage—areas where animals are prepared for euthanasia and areas where their bodies are stored afterward—has similar potential to undermine desired impressions. Precautions are thus taken to limit knowledge of the back stage and prevent the entry of outsiders. Private spaces are protected from public observance by doors, curtains, locks, and "Employees Only" signs. Sometimes outsiders are allowed into a few unauthorized areas but only in controlled circumstances such as visiting hours in the CCU. Guests must be guided by an escort who has the responsibility of signaling to fellow workers the proximity of outsiders and, hence, the need for cautious talk.

In addition to locked doors that hide the reality of backstage procedures, language is used to disguise procedures such as autopsies: "We have to get their permission to do an autopsy, but it is best not to be specific as to what an autopsy involves. You usually use the word *complete*, without getting graphic. You want to be careful about how those things are phrased." To make the reality of body storage more palatable for outsiders, veterinarians borrow from the euphemistic language of human body storage:

> We have our little morgue, which is the freezer. We never say it is the freezer to owners. We call it the morgue. It is not like the morgue on *Quincy* where they have their own little shelves. You may go in there and it looks like something out of [*The*] *Godfather* with a horse or sometimes, well, just a horse head. [*Laughs.*] Monday morning there may be a pile of bodies and dogs with their heads cut off [necessary for rabies detection], but owners don't need to know that. We don't, obviously, let them see that area. If they ask where the bodies go, I just say they go to our morgue.

Though most clinics hope that clients find solace in the nondescript but familiar language of morticians, some clinics couch the room in much less gloomy terms by calling it a groom room, implying that it is a place where animals are groomed rather than stored after death.

Naturally, veterinarians are sensitive to the fact that knowledge of these spaces could upset outsiders. Dr. Mulford described how she takes special precautions to maintain strict separation from backstage activities and hide certain realities from clients:

> In several of the clinics that I worked [in] you would have to walk past the waiting room [carrying a dead animal in a garbage bag] to the room where the freezer was [located]. Some people [other veterinarians] might walk by and say, "Oh, well, the owners don't know what's in [the bag] anyways." Which I guess is true; I guess they could just assume that it's garbage, that someone is taking out regular trash, but I'm always more cautious to make sure that people aren't going to see me with [the bags]. Just because I know it was sort of bothersome to me to discover that Fluffy, your beloved cat of fourteen years, is in a

Hefty garbage bag. [*Nervous laugh.*] I guess I'm always a little worried that someone's gonna see that and be like, "Oh my gosh, that's someone's pet."

Similarly, veterinarians would never place an animal in a body bag in front of clients: "The owner knows that no one is going to sit there with their dead pet till it gets cremated. They know that is going to happen, but they don't really want to be reminded of it. They don't want to think about what exactly happens to the body."

Even though the specifics of the backstage region are a mystery to most people, much of the time outsiders actively participate in maintaining the boundaries separating the back stage from the front. Most outsiders rarely express interest in the workings of the backstage area, and those who occasionally make inquires are generally satisfied with the vague answers typically offered to them by the veterinarian. Occasionally an owner will push for more detailed information, and the veterinarian must carefully consider word choice: "I have had some people push me about what we do with the body afterwards while they are waiting to be sent off to cremation, and I just try and brush it off." Most veterinarians recognize that separation of stages, or spheres, is integral to creating a satisfactory experience for pet owners.

With strict separation of spheres the veterinarian is most easily able to control desired impressions; however, the less distinct the front stage is from the back stage, the more difficult it is for the veterinarian to control the process. A fluid environment such that the activities of the back stage are close enough to interfere with the activities of the front stage can have serious consequences:

Noise from other animals barking in the background is kind of irritating because I really do want it to be peaceful and because it's stressful for the patient. Although most of the time the patient is not stressed out, but mostly it's stressful to the owner because of how they perceive it affects their patient. So, if it's a cat, the owner is going to be upset if there's fucking dogs barking, and when one dog is barking, it starts more dogs barking. . . . The problem for the staff is that we are so used to those sounds that we tune them out, . . . so often even when I ask them to [keep the dogs quiet], they don't do a very good job. . . . They aren't as conscious of it as they would be if they were in an otherwise quiet exam room trying to do a euthanasia with freaked-out owners and loud barking.

In some cases, veterinarians have no choice but to perform euthanasia in a backstage area because some patients are not stable enough to be moved from the critical wards. Because these euthanasia procedures take place directly in the back stage, the risk of offending behavior ruining a performance is highest.

Backstage wards are generally considered the least ideal locations for euthanasia because these spaces often foster impressions opposite those desired for euthanasia: "Euthanasia in the CCU sucks because there are techs running around doing things, treating other patients." Veterinarians typically loathe performing euthanasia procedures in the back stage: "It is a little uncomfortable to be standing there when people are just screaming and crying and wailing. You don't want the owners to feel like they are making a spectacle, even though they are. You want them to feel comfortable." Moreover, the veterinarian has less control over the environment:

> Another really bad thing is when people in the ICU are laughing or joking. I'll always warn all the techs [that I am doing a euthanasia in the ICU], but you can see there's a lot of staff on a busy day there, and there's a lot of shit going on. One time, I hadn't told the receptionist there was a euthanasia going on, so someone waltzed back there and loudly started talking about something totally inappropriate. And it was such an awful situation, and I was so helpless. I was literally right in the middle of the euthanasia, so I couldn't stop what I was doing to tell her to shut up.

Euthanasia procedures in the back stage can be complicated by the interference of backstage rhetoric. Unaware of the presence of outsiders, staff members' joking and laughing might disrupt the somber mood of the performance.

Setting the Mood in the Front Stage

When the environment is arranged to successfully separate the front stage from the back stage, the veterinarian is best able to control desired outcomes. Veterinary clinics and hospitals are increasingly building or converting examination rooms into rooms specifically designated for witness euthanasia. These meditation, comfort, memorial, or grieving rooms are designed to make the pet and the owner more comfortable and at ease. They are usually located in low-traffic areas of the hospital and, when possible, have a private exit so tearful clients can avoid going back through the public waiting area. Unlike sterile medical examination rooms, the walls are painted with soothing colors and are usually decorated with peaceful, scenic photos. They often have non-fluorescent, soft lighting and a supply of facial tissues, and they may also have plants or other greenery, a bowl with cat and dog treats, scissors for clipping fur, or clay for making memorial paw prints. The rooms are usually equipped with cozy seating and some may even have padded mats so owners can comfortably sit on the floor with their animals.

Allowing for the strongest separation of spheres, designated euthanasia rooms are preferred by many veterinarians. Without such rooms available, the veterinarian will choose a quiet examination room as far away from noise and distraction as possible. A private exit helps the veterinarian avoid potentially awkward interactions with grieving clients:

> After I euthanize a client's animal, I hate going into the hallway or the front and they see me laughing with another owner or a colleague or something. They are thinking, "Wow, that person wasn't affected at all by our euthanasia. That guy doesn't care. He has already forgotten about Max, and now he is laughing." That is not right for them to see me like that after euthanasia.

Participants fear such interactions may threaten their genuine expressions of empathy by leading clients to interpret their actions as insincere: "It can be weird if they see you turn right around and be all happy with another pet right after you euthanized their pet. That is something you just don't want them to see you doing."

Changing the sterile medical environment into a more intimate space not only enhances and personalizes the experience for the owner but also puts the veterinarian in the best position to control the client's impressions. Designated euthanasia spaces help veterinary actors achieve what Goffman calls "dramaturgical circumspection" by decreasing the risk of expected problems. In other words, the veterinarian will not have to work as hard for the audience to experience the event as peaceful, quiet, and tranquil. To that end, as more and more clients express a desire to be present during the death of their animals, many veterinary hospitals have invested in creating these specially designated euthanasia spaces.

While the right spaces and proper backstage preparation are critical to successful performances, the interactions with owners are where the performance needs final touches. In Goffman's dramaturgical model, social interaction is the most important part of the theatrical performance. The "actors" must work to consistently manage settings, clothing, words, and nonverbal actions to shape others' impressions. Fittingly, Goffman calls this "impression management."[16] An excerpt from my field notes shows how seriously veterinarians can take their role in impression management during euthanasia:

> While the novice veterinarian was euthanizing her first patient, she noticed that the dog had maggots living in an open wound and they were crawling over her hand. She wanted to run screaming from the room to express her disgust but could not do so, she said, *because* it was a euthanasia. Had it not been a euthanasia, she said that she might not have "freaked out," but she would have reacted differently. Instead, she managed to *conceal her actual feelings* from the owner. However, almost immediately after leaving the room, she vomited.

This veterinarian's successful performance depended on her ability to hide her disgust from the client. Goffman refers to a performer's ability to maintain a consistent performance, especially in the face of challenges, as having "dramaturgical discipline."[17] Like all good actors, veterinarians often act with the intent to conceal information from the audience that could damage the overall performance.

Many professions demand certain attitudes on the part of their workers through unofficial rules about the kinds of emotions that are (and are not) appropriate to express at work. Inspired by Arlie Hochschild's work in how workers are expected to evoke, suppress, or transform their emotion to meet the "feeling norms" of their occupation,[18] researchers have noted how workers in many occupations must hide or transform their emotions for others to see them as competent and to perform the requirements of their job.[19] For example, a nurse who panics at the sight of blood is of little use in an emergency room. Prison officers must push aside emotions of anger, disgust, anxiety, fear, pity, and sensitivity to deal coolly and dispassionately with dangerous inmates and threatening situations.[20] Workers are also expected to shift their emotions according to different contexts or interactions with different people.[21] For example, police officers are expected to convey negative emotions to suspected criminals and warmth to victims.[22] Similarly, veterinarians are expected to be cheerful service providers during standard checkups and somber, empathetic caregivers during euthanasia.

If veterinarians are consistently unable to effectively manage audience impressions, they may experience what Goffman terms a "spoiled identity."[23] Any actor's performance is, of course, subject to what is known in the theater as breaking character. Performers may act out of character by accident (if in the front stage) or on purpose (usually in the back stage). When a person accidentally breaks character, others try to ignore the performance flaw, such as when someone passes gas, trips over something, or spits when they speak. Just as an animal's physical reactions can mar the ideal euthanasia, so can the veterinarian's faulty presentation. Veterinarians have three major challenges to their dramaturgical discipline during euthanasia: a faulty presentation of their emotions, a rushed appearance, and seeming robotic or rehearsed.

Disciplined performers have the ability to disguise their spontaneous emotions when necessary. Hiding emotions, if they are not congruent with desired impressions, is often considered essential to a good performance. According to Arlie Hochschild's concept, veterinarians do "emotional labor" by carefully monitoring their own expressions of emotions during euthanasia performances.[24] Displays of anger, for example, are especially important to suppress (albeit difficult):

> I was so mad at them because his diabetes was really unregulated, and they obviously did not make the necessary efforts to care for him. . . . I feel like with euthanasia, though, when we are angry with them, it is not the right time to show it. . . . I would not have wanted to do that euthanasia because I was really annoyed at them. It would have been a challenge to be sympathetic.

Sometimes veterinarians are shocked by owner behavior or think it weird:

> The thing that really was the most shocking thing for me . . . is when they want to take pictures with the animal before and after death. . . . I was completely unprepared for that whole phenomenon of pictures of the dead body. . . . Someone wanted to take a picture of me and their dead dog. Several times people have wanted me to take pictures during and after the euthanasia. That is really weird. Why would you want pictures of your dog being put to sleep? I don't understand. It is the most disturbing thing I have ever experienced—ever. I try to act like I am okay and it is normal, but it is a very, very strange request.

One novice intern had a concern that he would not be able to keep his emotions under control during his first euthanasia: "My first one, well, *all* I am going to be thinking about is trying not to cry. Man, I really hope I don't cry."

Sometimes veterinarians have to guard against the temptation to laugh during euthanasia. In one such case, a husband and wife were fighting over what to do with the body of their dog. The wife wanted to bury him in the same plot as her father because the dog had once belonged to him, but the husband didn't think it possible, given that her father had been dead for a few years. The husband said, "You can't bury the dog in the cemetery; they won't let you." And the wife replied, "I'm going to do it anyway, Henry. I'll go there at night, and you'll come with me, won't you?" Henry sarcastically agreed, "Yeah, yeah; I'll come with you at night and bury the dog. I'll come with you with my mask and flashlight and bust into the cemetery and bury the dog." After Meredith made it known she was displeased with her husband's sarcasm, his anger came out, "Damn it, Meredith! You can't even plant a flower without permission; why do you think they're going to let you bury the dog?" Both the veterinarian and I found it particularly challenging not to laugh at such a strange argument.

Laughter is rarely considered appropriate in euthanasia but can be difficult to stifle. Sometimes a client will have an emotional reaction that catches the veterinarian off guard. These reactions can be touching but also funny, such as when a big, gruff man begins to sob uncontrollably:

> I may have a nurse in the room with me and we will be totally dead serious while this man is sobbing. . . . He went from this man who you would think had never cried in his life to a little child who is just wailing. You are all serious in the room, and you pat his shoulder, and you say I am so sorry, and you tell him to take some time. . . . .You walk into the ICU, and you and the nurse look at each other, and you just fucking crack up, and it is not funny [*laughs*], but you know how unexpected things can be humorous? . . . It is things like that that are just fucking humorous.

The incongruity between the reaction the veterinarian expected and the actual, reverse reaction may spark laughter for veterinary staff. Sometimes unplanned events by the animal during euthanasia can be experienced as humorous:

> There are horrible things that can be kind of funny, like maybe an animal falls in an awkward position, and you are thinking, "Oh shit, that didn't just happen." They might have, like, blowout diarrhea, and that is horrible but [*laughs*] can be, in a way, funny. Yet in the privacy of the ICU, away from the owner and away from the sanctity of that room, some acts are hilarious, and you have to vent, because sometimes it is so awful that it is funny.

Unusual client behavior has a similar effect: "There was this one lady with her cat, and all of a sudden she just broke out into this—I think it was some kind of Latin song or prayer, and she just kept, like, chanting over and over again. . . . I kind of bit my tongue a little bit because, honestly, it was hard not to laugh. It's awful to say, but sometimes you are just so uncomfortable it is hard not to laugh."

Laughing, although it does break the somber mood, does not always ruin a performance. Owners, for example, sometimes make statements intending to be amusing or tell a funny story about their animal. The veterinarian often responds with a comical retort. For example, during the euthanasia of a particularly feisty dog known to bite, an owner commented while simultaneously laughing and crying, "That dog was a real jerk. He will probably bite dogs in heaven." Dr. Shelly responded in kind, "Well, you know that dog across the ward is relieved, because he hated him, and we all know how much he wanted to bite him." When unsure if the client is open to humor, participants often look to cues from clients:

> You just try to not laugh when certain things go wrong, like when you fart or an owner farts or the dog farts. [*Laughs.*] Most of the owners will . . . laugh along with you, especially when the animal is doing something funny—you might as well laugh. You kind of follow the owners' lead. You don't want to be the one laughing while they are crying. If they chuckle, then I feel a little bit better about chuckling too.

Although they respond appropriately to clients' jokes, veterinarians typically do not laugh or make comic statements unless the owner does first.

Euthanasia can be sad for veterinarians, particularly when the veterinarian has known the pet for a long time or has invested significant efforts to make the animal well again. The outward expression of sadness is not necessarily considered problematic, although most veterinarians try to limit their public display of sadness, as Dr. Edwards explained:

> I am supposed to be the one who does this every day. . . . I am okay if I am teary-eyed and they aren't, but I don't want to be unable to have some composure and be able to speak when I need to talk. I don't want to be like having to blow my nose while they are just sitting over there watching me euthanize their pet. It just doesn't seem appropriate to show more emotion than they do even if I feel pretty attached to their animal. You don't want to get to the point where you are making the client uncomfortable 'cause you are crying. I think that there is a certain point that you can let yourself get to and then you need to then check it.

Even when veterinarians do not feel a special bond with the owners or their animal, they can unexpectedly feel sadness and an uncontrollable desire to cry: "Remember the one where the woman told her dog that she missed her already? You lost it a little and so did I, but I really tried not to cry. That one was sad. It is hard not to lose it sometimes, but it feels really weird when you are crying and you just met this owner and this animal a few minutes ago."

While some presentations required veterinarians to mask or tone down their emotions, at other ones participants felt the need to express emotions they were not experiencing. For example, the desired emotions of compassion and sympathy can be difficult to deliver:

I used to watch that show *Six Feet Under*, and I imagine[d] what it must be like for funeral directors, because they are always expected to feel sympathy for the family or at least look like they are sad. There is only so much of that you can maintain day after day. For me it comes and goes, but I can sure identify with them on the issue. I always feel something, but some days more than others . . . you make the effort to transition into that mode if you are not there yourself. I could be joking around with a friend right before I walk into the room, but as soon as I walk in, I change immediately.

Dr. Madfis explained, "Euthanasia is different because you need to have compassion at all times while you are doing it. You need to show it even if you don't really feel it, like if you are tired and it is your tenth one today or whatever. It is the owner's first one of the day—and maybe of their lives. You have to be sympathetic looking even if you were just arguing with them five minutes ago."

If the veterinarian fears he or she might not be able to properly manage emotional expression, seeking another veterinarian to perform the euthanasia can circumvent potential failure. By asking another veterinarian to do a difficult euthanasia, the veterinarian is practicing Goffman's "dramaturgical circumspection." Veterinarians often rely on other team members to aid in successful presentations, and sometimes even a complete replacement as a last resort. However, when actors work together successfully as team members, they are said to have "dramaturgical loyalty." Dr. Miller described the importance of trusting her teammates to help each other maintain dramaturgical discipline:

Our nurses are awesome, and I know they feel the same way I do, and they are going to wait until we get into the ICU [to laugh or express inappropriate emotions], and they are going to keep their voices down. The kind that might make a comment on the way out the door—I won't even have them close to me. I will make it really clear that it is not cool to be so careless around owners. I will give them the look of death. It is so unacceptable to me. Those are things that you have to be aware of so they are not giving the wrong impression either. . . . It is really my pet peeve, and I will not work with . . . a nurse or another doctor who I don't trust to have some tact.

Although team members work together to maintain dramaturgical discipline, some can carelessly or mistakenly disrupt a euthanasia and threaten the veterinarian's dramaturgical discipline.

Euthanasia performances are considered ruined if the veterinarian appears rushed, thus a second major challenge to veterinarians' presentation of self is when they are particularly busy: "Definitely in regular exams I will be very different and much more efficient. I will sometimes cut people off and try to make them hurry. With euthanasia I am more relaxed and open to their needs and I let them talk even when they go on and on." Veterinarians want to give the impression that they are taking their time, especially during euthanasia: "I have a different tone and speed. I speak quietly during euthanasia and I try to give the impression I am doing things slowly and carefully." Participants wanted owners to feel free to take as much time as they desired before, during, and after the euthanasia: "In most exams we try and control everything from the conversation on. We control the direction. We control the pace. We control what happens, but with the euthanasia you let them run the show. This can be very difficult on a busy shift."

Ideally, euthanasia is scheduled during a time when the veterinarian is not booked with other appointments or surgeries, but this is not always possible. Then veterinarians have to pretend they are not rushed: "If you have critical patients waiting . . . you are trying not to rush it, but you are trying to rush it. It is hard when you don't have the time to really sit in there for a few minutes. If you don't have the time, you have to make it seem like you have the time." Thus, a nice feature of the new euthanasia rooms is that they give clients a private space where they will not be disturbed, freeing the veterinarian to attend to other duties and to simply check in every so often. Veterinarians must strike a balance between efficiency and spending enough time with owners to foster desired impressions.

Performances are considered ruined if clients interpret the veterinarian's actions as rehearsed, cold, or robotic. Veterinarians establish patterns to help avoid technical error, but they run the risk of becoming too rigid in their routines:

I have my way of doing euthanasia so it goes smooth[ly], and I wouldn't say it's rehearsed, but I'm so used to saying the speech I give. And I feel like it helps me too. . . . I don't call it ritualistic but . . . when something in the ritual is out of step, it makes you feel uncomfortable. Or if the owners try to push to the next step before you're ready, you think, "No, no, we [have] got to do this first, then this, then this." You create this pattern because you don't want it to be uncomfortable for anyone . . . but you have to be flexible so you don't come off as a robot.

Dr. Eggerman agreed: "Everyone is different and their relationship with their pet is different, so you are tailoring the standard process to the individual. I do special things because I don't want it to seem like a machine. They don't want to feel like a cog in the machine and [that] the death of their animal is just routine to me. They want you to notice their animal is unique."

Some veterinarians always disdain money collection or paperwork, while others worry that these unsavory tasks when related to euthanasia procedures made them seem cold or heartless. For the veterinarian, these impersonal acts of business have the potential to ruin the desired impression of euthanasia as a caring and personal act:

I am *not* taking a credit card from someone if I am about to kill something. . . . When the decision is made with me during an exam, I ask someone from the front desk to take care of that stuff for me. . . . Sometimes the decision is made in an emergency, and in those cases I tell them to walk right past the desk and go home. I say that we will bill you, and I will take the heat for it, but I never really get in trouble for it because these people usually do pay. I try to avoid at all costs any sort of formal or administrative interaction after they have watched their pet die.

Delegating bureaucratic tasks to receptionists allowed veterinarians to separate themselves as medical professionals from the impersonal acts of paperwork and money collection. When delegation was not possible, tackling bureaucratic issues before the euthanasia ensured that the intimacy so carefully fostered during euthanasia was not broken down afterward.

Providing owners with choices for customizing their euthanasia experience leaves clients feeling that their unique relationship to their pet was recognized by the veterinarian: "What they want is what we do, and we should make it clear that they have options. The dog can be standing on the floor [for the euthanasia] or . . . on a blanket or . . . in their lap, or they might want to lie on the floor next to him. We do whatever is going to make you and the dog the most comfortable." Veterinarians often go the extra mile for their clients during euthanasia:

> I ask if they want me to bring chairs, blankets, or pillows or if they want me to bring them some water or a cup of coffee or a last meal for their pet. I've literally listed menus before. I was like "We have chicken, and we have tuna. We have a food called AD, and it is for anorexic animals—it's delicious." If [pets] like kibble, we have all sorts of kibble. I can bring them a little buffet. I'll bring them a plate of different foods and just let them gorge themselves, if they're still eating. No request is too much . . . not when it comes to euthanasia.

Dr. Yang described feeding animals a last meal of their favorite food:

> This dog, his favorite thing was cheese, so I went back to the hole [intern office] and got some string cheese. And the owners went to the little vending machines and got everything they knew he always liked, like an ice-cream sandwich and a hot pocket and chips. And the dog ate gung ho in the room. And they hung out with him for most of the night, just kind of feeding him and talking with him. And I stopped by, and they showed me pictures and shared stories, and they were there for a good four hours. But it was so good.

Decisions about who will attend the euthanasia are typically left up to the owners. Sometimes this may mean that whole families—including children, friends, and neighbors—come in for euthanasia. "Because it is, like, their last moment, no request is excessive. . . . I've had thirteen people in a room. . . . And I just squeeze between people." Veterinarians may also make special exceptions to hospital policies for euthanasia:

> I never allow owners to hold their animals for vaccinations and such, but you try to make exceptions for euthanasia. Cats in particular are epinephrine driven, and lots of things can set them off. They may freak out and bite the owner. If they want to have the animal on their lap, it would depend on the demeanor of the animal. If it is a fifteen-year-old cat who is old, sick, and quiet, I probably would let them. From a liability standpoint, lawyers would tell you never ever, ever let the client hold the animal for anything because if they get hurt, they

will sue you. That is a judgment call. An old, sick, friendly golden retriever that has lymphoma I would let the people put . . . on their lap. It may get excited and bite them, but that is a judgment call.

For the convenience of the client or comfort of the patient, euthanasia may be done in the owner's car or outside the hospital in a grassy area. One veterinarian explained:

> We ended up taking the dog outside. I suggested we take him outside and sat out under a tree over in the corner. . . . And [in] some of the stories she had told me when we had been talking a little bit, she had talked about how he used to go hiking. He'd recently been up to New Hampshire with them on a nice hike. And when we talked about it and signed the papers, they were going to take the body to New Hampshire with them, and that's where they were going next to bury him. And so I asked her if she wanted to go outside, and then we did and took a blanket and went outside. And the dog was, he was slow, but he meandered out on his own. When he got out, he tried to sit on his owner, which made everybody laugh. And we let him go, and I got the most amazing letter from them. [*Crying.*] They were so thankful.

Although not always possible or practical, a few participants offered to perform the procedure in an owner's home or under a favorite tree in their yard: "I really like the idea of at home euthanasia with a terminal animal. The owners love it, and it is pleasant and dignified, and people are really happy about it." Home euthanasia is offered only in rare circumstances, as it is time consuming and the veterinarian is left without backup medical supplies and technical support.

In response to clients' desires to be with their companion animals when they die, veterinarians are increasingly concerned with creating the experience of a peaceful death of the animal for their human clients. Because of the impossibility of redoing euthanasia in the event of mistakes, the veterinarian must attend to its performance aspects. Veterinarians recognize the importance of showmanship with euthanasia and work to create successful performances:

> You have to put on a show really. It is not like you are acting but you have to have a specific tone about you. It can *feel* like a performance though. . . . Your inflections go down when you are trying to convey

something more melancholy. You can totally feel it right when you go into the room. The air is different. You change the way you act and the way you talk, and you are aware of the way you look and what your eyes are doing and your body language is doing. When I am talking to owners and getting a history [during everyday examinations], I am standing or doing other things all at once, but when I am talking about euthanasia, I am always at their level. If they are on the floor, I am with them and touching their pet and trying to demonstrate to them in some way that this is not insignificant. . . . In that sense it is a lot of extra work.

Although many novice veterinarians are quite anxious about their lack of experience interacting with clients during euthanasia, nearly all learn how to host successful performances:

I have gotten good at doing it [euthanasia] well. I guess it sounds sort of heartless, but I feel like I have developed the right things to say and what not to say. I think I have gotten a very good feel for what works and what doesn't work. All of my euthanasia experiences go very smoothly now. I know which animals I have to put IV catheters in and which ones I can just stick in the room, and I know how much time to give owners. It is all sort of a sixth sense that I have developed about people and euthanasia. You just learn this through the experience of the years. I have gotten good at that, and I know that it is as valuable a service as giving a vaccine. I have gotten a good routine down, and I do a *good presentation.* (Emphasis added)

While each veterinarian develops a core set of routines to help guarantee successful euthanasia experiences, he or she also tries to remain flexible enough to fit an individual client's needs and wishes.

Goffman's dramaturgical metaphor becomes an interpretive framework that illuminates the meaning and function embedded in everyday social interactions, aspects of our lives we might mistakenly overlook as mere social protocol or trivial etiquette. Separating the front- and backstage areas allows the veterinarian to better control the performance. The veterinarian's interactional rituals provide stability and predictability for clients and help limit the potential for disorder and uncertainty for the veterinarian. Failed performances, veterinarians fear, could cost their professional relationship with the client, thus effective staging of the show helps guard against mistakes and leads the audience to a favorable impression of the veterinarian.

Scholars debate the dynamics of impression management and the motivations of actors. Some sociologists argue that actors use impression-management strategies primarily for profit,[25] while others argue that the actor does not always seek to control impression for calculated advantage.[26] Within the dramaturgical framework, it is not difficult to interpret actors as scheming and manipulating to deceive others for their own benefit (perhaps especially for profit motives). Jason Ulsperger and John Paul examine impression-management techniques of workers in for-profit nursing homes to shape positive images of the care offered.[27] Fortunetellers use backstage deceptions to control the perceptions of potential clients and exploit them for profit.[28]

Veterinarians, unlike funeral directors, are not in the business of death, and their income is not directly dependent on euthanasia performances. However, veterinarians advertise grieving rooms on their clinic's web page, perhaps as a marketing tool designed to attract new customers. Many clinics sell memorial jewelry or containers designed for storing clippings of a pet's hair or an ink print of their paw. Veterinarians, like funeral directors, take on the responsibility of dealing with the remains of the deceased, providing their own cremation services or contracting with commercial venders. If the owners wish to keep their pet's ashes, they can purchase one of several styles of memorial urns. If they wish to take the animal's body home for burial, veterinarians may offer disposable coffin-shaped cardboard boxes or handcrafted wooden pet caskets from commercial venders. In general, however, veterinary clinics make very little profit from these items.

Euthanasia procedures are often time-consuming, and veterinarians make very little profit from them. Moreover, they will no longer be able to earn money from treating the animals they euthanize. Despite this, veterinarians increasingly argue that successful euthanasia experiences contribute to financial success. In a lecture to third-year veterinary students, Professor Allen stressed the importance of successful euthanasia performances for building long-term relationships with clients:

> When I graduated from vet school . . . one of the first things a vet told me was, "You know, Ray, there is only one thing that you need to do well as a veterinarian." I said, "What is that?" He said, "How to eu-thanize an animal. . . . If you can euthanize an animal well, gracefully, and with respect and compassion, when they [clients] go home and have that visceral response, they will think, 'My God. I really *love* my veterinarian. He really understands how I feel.' Even though it was a negative experience or an extremely emotional experience, they will

feel that way. They absolutely will remember that compassion when their future pets need services."

Impression management in veterinary euthanasia is multifaceted. Dramatizing and ritualizing euthanasia procedures has many benefits for the client and veterinarian alike. For example, properly staging the euthanasia avoids mistakes for the veterinarian, but it also adds weight and significance to the event for the client. The amount of effort veterinary staff put into the death of the animal reinforces the notion that the companion animal was valuable and significant to both clients and colleagues. By memorializing and ritualizing an animal's death, veterinarians demonstrate that the animal was valuable, worthy of such honor, ceremony, and human grief. Of course, by extension, such acts of veneration also serve as a sign that companion animals are worth the cost of expensive medical care, a point not lost even on the least-business-savvy veterinarian.

3

Strange Intimacy

Managing Pet Owners' Emotions

oday's companion-animal veterinarians not only attend to the death of their animal patients; they must also deal with emotionally distraught clients before and after they have made the difficult decision to end the life of their companion animal. As seen in Chapter 2, veterinarians work to manage pet owners' impressions of their animal's death such that they have a good last memory of their animal and think of euthanasia as a positive experience. In addition to managing owners' impressions, veterinarians consider managing their emotions important to the creation of an overall good death, a successful euthanasia. Yet allowing owners to witness the euthanasia of their animals (fittingly described as witness euthanasia by some veterinarians) is a fairly new practice in veterinary medicine.

As a profession, veterinary medicine has only relatively recently involved the lives (and deaths) of pet animals. Until the middle of the twentieth century, veterinarians were almost exclusively charged with maintaining the optimal physical condition of economically valuable transportation and farm animals.[1] Before the mid-twentieth century, pet owners often diagnosed, treated, and nursed their own sick animals at home.[2] Early pet owners cared for their pets' health and well-being, and when it came to ending the lives of suffering or unwanted animals, they did that at home. While some companion animals were left to die on their own, others were killed by their owners. Over time, however, pet owners began to perceive home methods such as shooting or drowning as inconvenient, distasteful, and in some cases, cruel or inhumane.[3] Though shooting animals was considered a humane method of euthanizing farm pets at the time, for example, audiences watching one of the most memorable scenes in cinema today feel for the young man in the film *Old Yeller* who must shoot and kill his beloved, but potentially rabid, dog. Some urban pet owners, often without access to firearms, began to overdose their animals with the anesthetic chloroform, an expensive but more aesthetic method of killing. Concerned with how best to alleviate (or simply evaluate) their animals' suffering, pet owners progressively turned to veterinarians for assistance—not only in managing their pets' health but in attending to their deaths as well.

Euthanasia became an increasingly common task for modern veterinarians and typically took place in the backrooms of clinics, far from the view of pet owners. As late as 1981, articles in veterinary journals strongly discouraged client access to the death of their pets out of concern that witnessing the death of beloved companions might be emotionally disturbing for clients and an additional time-consuming burden for practitioners.[4] While some old-line veterinarians still ban pet owners from witnessing euthanasia procedures, many of today's veterinarians criticize such policy as old-fashioned and inconsiderate of clients' desires and expectations. Surveys of veterinarians and clients found that between 70 and 77 percent of respondents strongly believe a veterinarian should provide the option to clients to be present during euthanasia.[5] However, from a veterinarian's perspective, the presence of a pet owner can bring additional challenges in terms of managing the owner's impressions of the pet death and attending to the bereaved's emotional needs.

Inspired by Arlie Hochschild's groundbreaking work on emotions, scientific interest in occupational groups' management (evoking, suppressing, or transforming) of the emotions of others has increased in recent years.[6] For example, scholars have uncovered how physicians influence the emotions of ordinary patients,[7] patients labeled problematic,[8] patients with serious illness,[9] and even the emotions of patients' grieving families.[10] In a variety of other workplace settings, researchers have noted the ways workers use emotion-management strategies to achieve interactional and organizational goals.[11] For example, search-and-rescue workers count on emotion-management strategies to make interactions with tearful family members and distressed victims less likely to happen and less awkward when they do.[12] Bill collectors are taught to manipulate debtors' emotions to recover their employers' revenue—an obvious organizational goal.[13]

Emotion is a private, internal sensation, and accurately perceiving another's feelings can be difficult. One obvious way people allow others access to their inner feelings is to describe them; however, individuals seldom directly state their emotions. For example, victims aided by search-and-rescue volunteers in Jennifer Lois's study rarely directly stated, "I feel embarrassed"; nonetheless, rescue workers commonly identified and managed this emotion during rescue attempts.[14] Of course, though workers may label other people's feelings (e.g., regret, joy, fear, anger, or sorrow), there is little guarantee that their interpretations are accurate. Yet Linda Francis argues that the open discussion of feelings is often not necessary for an emotional exchange, because individuals permit others access to their emotions through what she terms "interpersonal emotion management" when they allow them to direct, mold, induce, or alter their emotions.[15] Although a fascinating topic, I do not deal explicitly with veterinarians' interpretation of others' emotions in this chapter; instead, I consider their response to the perceived emotions of their clients.

What follows next is a description of the major types of emotions expressed by pet owners and the respective management strategies of veterinarians. In this chapter, I detail veterinarians' reliance on emotion-management techniques applied to the emotions of their human clients, specifically grief and guilt. Next, I discuss the affective role veterinarians assume in comforting bereaved pet owners and how that role initiates an unexpected gratitude response from pet owners. To explain this unique finding, I explore how societal attitudes regarding nonhuman animals shape veterinarian-client relationships.

Pet Owners' Emotions: Guilt and Grief

Unlike the ordinary, unemotional veterinary consultation, euthanasia-related conversations between the veterinarian and client are often marked by at least some degree of emotional distress.[16] Although I witnessed some seemingly callous decisions by pet owners regarding the death of their animals, I more often witnessed emotionally distraught owners who asked to hold their companion animals during the euthanasia and spend time with their bodies after they died (with the deaths of not just dogs and cats but also birds, mice, ferrets, hamsters, and even an iguana). While some pet owners self-labeled their feelings, participants described a wide range of emotions they believe clients express. However, for the most part participants classified their clients' emotions into two main categories: those associated with grief (e.g., sadness, distress, and tears) and those associated with guilt (e.g., doubt and regret).

How clients experience grief[17] and guilt[18] over the death of a companion animal is influenced by factors such as the length of pet ownership, circumstances of death, and level of emotional attachment. However, research suggests the deaths of companion animals have increasingly become significant stressors in the lives of pet owners.[19] Although the experience of grief varies from pet owner to pet owner, for many, the death of a companion animal is a highly emotional experience that is just as devastating as the loss of a human signifi-cant other.[20] In Geraldine Gage and Ralph Holcomb's study, males rated pet loss as about as stressful as the loss of a close friendship, while females rated it as about as stressful as losing touch with their married children.[21] Researchers find similar grief reactions from people mourning the death of animals and from those who experience human loss.[22] Thomas Wrobel and Amanda Dye's study of adults whose pet had recently died found that 86 percent initially experienced at least one symptom of grief, 35 percent at six months, and 22 percent at one year.[23]

The decision to end the life of a companion animal can intensify the grief process and cause many pet owners to experience guilt.[24] Some pet owners feel guilt for merely considering giving consent for euthanasia, and others report feelings of guilt and failure long after the animal's death.[25] For example, a decision to euthanize based primarily on financial reasons or resulting from a medical problem that the client allowed to go unattended can weigh heav-ily on a pet owner's mind, causing significant feelings of regret and guilt.[26] Clients even expressed guilt for circumstances they had no influence over, such as an animal developing cancer. They may assume responsibility for the death of the animal because of not asking enough questions or not getting another opinion before deciding on euthanasia.

Cindy Adams, Brenda Bonnett, and Alan Meek found that although most respondents to their survey believed euthanasia was a humane option, approximately half felt guilty about their decision or questioned whether they had made the right decision.[27] Pet owners, concerned about their choice to euthanize, often ruminate about the timing of euthanasia and may phone their veterinarians after their pet's death seeking reassurance that their choice to end their pet's life was reasonable, appropriate, and in their pet's best inter-est.[28] For example, some clients of my study's participants thought they should have delayed longer before deciding on euthanasia, while others thought they might have waited too long and the animal suffered. A few clients even felt guilt that the strength and intensity of their emotions was greater over their animal's death than for the loss of a human relationship.

To manage their clients' guilt and grief, veterinarians relied on different strategies before and after the euthanasia, a finding congruent with studies showing that workers strategically apply emotion management techniques as dictated by contextual demands. For example, when studying search-and-rescue staff, Jennifer Lois found that they manage the emotions of victims in qualitatively different ways from how they manage family members' emotions.[29] In other words, the targeted emotion work of rescuers allows for the successful rescue of distressed victims in one context and lessens the awkwardness of tearful interactions with family members in another context. Drawing on Erving Goffman's insights, Lois describes how rescue workers *tightly* control victims' emotions and create *loose* emotional guidelines for family members. In *Behavior in Public Places* Goffman argues that all social situations are marked by a certain degree of "tightness" or "looseness": in "tight occasions . . . the participants have many onerous situational obligations, and [in] loose occasions . . . [they are] relatively free of these constraints."[30] When interacting with family members desperately awaiting news of their missing or endangered loved ones, rescue workers allow family members to cathartically "express a variety of emotions related to their grief, such as guilt or joy about the past, uncertainty or faith about the present, and fear or hope about the future."[31] Rescue workers create loose emotional situations for anxious families by holding them to relatively few behavioral and emotional obligations. However, to rescue distressed victims, workers need to construct rigid, or tight, behavioral and emotional expectations for them.

During rescue situations, workers "wield a great deal of authority in defining the situation and, thus, the norms and roles that correspond to it. They establish power by taking control and demanding specific emotional reactions from others, from whom they allow little input."[32] Rescue workers tightly manage emotion because certain emotions interfere with rescue attempts. For example, tight emotion work helps victims save face when embarrassed regarding their predicament and remain focused when they feel anxious during the rescue. Thus workers tightly transform and suppress unwanted emotions in the rescue context, but they loosely manage the emotions of family, allowing the open expression of vulnerable emotions. The targeted emotion-management strategies of rescue workers help both family members and victims "arrive at particularly healthy and useful emotions for their situation."[33] I apply Lois's findings in this chapter to explore how veterinarians strategically apply emotion-management techniques as dictated by contextual demands and interactional goals.

Managing Guilt: Veterinarians' Use of Tight Emotion Management

The question of when it is appropriate to euthanize a patient can be a complicated and emotional matter for the veterinarian. Hours can feel like days for veterinarians who believe that an animal is suffering but the owner is unable to decide on the course to take. One such case involved a feline patient who had been struck by a car and suffered serious but treatable injuries. The owner could not afford the emergency fee—let alone the amount necessary to save his cat—but he clearly did not want to end his companion's life. After administering pain medication to the cat, Dr. Dever desperately tried to convince the client to authorize surgery or euthanasia. Explaining her frustration to me, Dr. Dever firmly believes her client's emotions prevented him from making a difficult choice for the animal's welfare: "This man is suffering from serious grief at the thought of losing his cat, but he also feels guilty because he let her get outside the house. . . . You can't waffle on something like this. They need to be euthanized or treated. You saw this cat's tail was degloved [the skin torn back in a manner similar to taking off a glove]. It is inhumane to leave this animal the way it is, and it can be agonizing on us when they won't make that decision."

In animal emergency rooms, where patients who have consumed rat poison or been struck by a car wait, every moment can count, and veterinarians often experience a significant amount of frustration, tension, and stress if clients do not make timely decisions. In urgent cases, the client's emotions (particularly guilt and grief) may impair ability to make timely medical decisions or even lead to bad decisions. Thus, the veterinarian's goals are typically instrumental—helping assuage clients' emotions so they can make rational, emotion-free choices.

Circumstances in which guilt is not easily managed are often particularly frustrating for the veterinarian, as demonstrated by the case of Daisy, a golden retriever who swallowed a toothpick accidentally left inside her owner's hamburger. When the toothpick perforated her gastrointestinal tract, she developed debilitating peritonitis. After Daisy's first surgery to correct the damage, she relapsed. Because of the severity of her condition, the intern strongly recommended euthanasia. However, Daisy's owner responded, "I can't kill her. It is my fault she ate the toothpick. I have to give her another chance." Unable to change the client's mind, the intern reluctantly agreed to another surgery. After three weeks in intensive care and two major surgeries, the peritonitis returned. Despite a bill spiraling past $10,000 and the surgeon's prediction that Daisy would likely not survive another surgery, the client wanted to try again. Concerned another surgery would cause Daisy unnecessary suffering, a supervisor called the intern into her office to discuss the mounting bill and the owner's refusal to euthanize. The intern, clearly frustrated with the situation, loudly exclaimed, "What do you want me to do? Put a gun to his head? He just feels too damn guilty over that fucking toothpick!"

To avoid outcomes like Daisy's, participants discouraged feelings of guilt by strictly requiring clients to conform to specific emotional directives, thus tightly managing clients' guilt. More specifically, they neutralized guilt by relying on a small selection of emotion-management strategies also observed in Vaughn DeCoster's study of physician-patient interaction: reinterpret, redirect, and rationalize.[34] Even when euthanasia seems irrefutably in the best interest of the animal, simply contemplating ending their animal's life can threaten clients' positive identity as good and loving pet owners. For these, veterinarians reinterpreted their clients' guilt in favor of more constructive emotions. For instance, one participant encouraged a client to reinterpret her guilt as love for the animal: "Lots of owners who choose euthanasia feel guilt and they doubt their decision, but that's just a sign of your love for Scratchers. It is not a sign that you are making a bad decision, but that you care deeply for Scratchers's best interest."

Veterinarians continue to tightly squash their client's feelings of guilt after the client makes the difficult decision to euthanize the companion animal. Participants often used the same strategies after euthanasia that they had previously relied on to facilitate timely decisions. For example, clients often felt guilty considering euthanasia for terminally ill patients because they feared they might be making the decision to euthanize their pets too soon. In response, participants redirected their client's guilt toward the animal's potential future pain. This strategy encouraged the client to focus on the negative emotions they would unquestionably feel in the future if they allowed the animal to needlessly suffer. However, even after the death of the animal, the veterinarian will often continue to redirect clients' expressions of guilt into concern for the animal's feelings. One veterinarian, for example, redirected her client's guilt by focusing on how her decision to euthanize ended the suffering of her treasured pet: "We did everything we possibly could, and at least she is not suffering anymore. No more chemo. No more needles. No more throwing up."

When clients felt guilty for merely thinking of euthanizing their pet, rationalizing was an especially helpful tactic in gaining the veterinarian's goal: helping owners make timely decisions. For instance, when Dr. Sanchez has concluded that the options to treat or euthanize are fairly equal for his patient, he tries to rationalize both options for his clients: "People can feel guilt by just considering euthanasia. Guilt gets in the way, so you have to make sure that they understand that both options are good. You just have to try and help them see some options through the guilt." Dr. Mulford made a similar comment about how she handles guilt being the largest obstacle to decision making:

> If both the option to treat and the option to euthanize are pretty
> equal—like, in my medical opinion, the case could go either way—I

just try and present the options equally. . . . The people that come in with a very sick animal—the big thing I will tell people a lot of the time is that these are the things we can do, but honestly you could have all the money in the world and I couldn't promise you that you would get back a healthy animal. On the other hand, if treatment is a medically reasonable option as well, you have to make both options equally appealing.

By rationalizing both options as legitimate, participants let clients know that they, trained experts, believed euthanasia was a legitimate option.

In the decision-making phase, veterinarians may rationalize euthanasia as only one justifiable outcome among other equally legitimate alternatives. Yet when the client chooses euthanasia, the veterinarian may shift position and rationalize the client's choice as the most legitimate. Consider a rottweiler named Spike. At first his veterinarian rationalized either euthanizing or continuing life-sustaining treatment: "Though Spike could certainly respond to the new treatments, twelve years old is really old for a rottweiler. It is obvious that you took really good care of him and gave him a great life, so I know, whichever decision you make, it's the right one." Yet after the client made the decision to euthanize Spike, the veterinarian exclusively rationalized his client's choice: "You did the right thing. . . . This was the right call in my opinion. Many people make the mistake of waiting too late. A big problem we run into is when people won't make timely decisions and the animal suffers. It is obvious that you love Spike and you didn't want him to suffer."

As Dr. Eggerman explained, veterinarians often rationalized their clients' choices even when they had hoped for a different outcome for their patient: "As long as [I] feel like [euthanasia] is somewhat medically justifiable . . . I will transition from having potentially—usually kind of tactfully—argued for the other side to supporting them and making them feel good about their decision." Dr. Kaufman described the transition she makes to help clients deal with guilt:

When they choose euthanasia, I immediately go from [a point] I've been arguing . . . to "I'm so sorry. I understand this must be really hard for you, and Fluffy is a great dog," even though technically I might have been totally opposed to it a minute ago. But all of a sudden you align yourself on their side. You have too. You cannot fucking hold a grudge. That's not fair to them. Regardless, it's a hard decision. And they brought their pet into a vet for a reason. They obviously care about the pet, so even if it is not the decision that you would make, it's their decision to make.

Thus, some participants validated and rationalized a client's choice even when that choice went against the outcome they desired for the patient.

Given that euthanasia procedures are technically simple procedures, I once asked a veterinarian why they do not rely on technicians to do them. Like several others whom I asked the same question, Dr. Garrett believed her clients would prefer a doctor to euthanize their animals because that role reinforces the legitimacy of the owners' choice to euthanize their animal:

> If it didn't matter to them, then why don't people drop their animals off at shelters to be euthanized? Why don't they go to a technical expert who does euthanasia all day long? Most people go to a veterinarian. They want a doctor to be there because the doctor gives their choice legitimacy and helps them feel okay with the choice. The doctor is able to validate their decision in a medical way or in a way that a technician just cannot do . . . socially speaking.

For many anxious pet owners, having the veterinarian corroborate the difficult decision to end their animal's life was often a great relief. As medical experts regarding animal health and well-being, veterinarians wield a great deal of authority in defining the best interest of animals. And participants often relied on this authority to tightly control the meaning of euthanasia as a positive, medically appropriate choice.

In their role as tight emotion managers, veterinarians strove to not only help clients resolve guilt but also shape euthanasia as a positive and loving option for animals. Participants so tightly controlled the meaning of euthanasia that they refused to allow any disparaging remarks from their clients regarding euthanasia. For example, in the following exchange recorded in my field notes, a veterinarian transformed her client's pessimistic statement regarding euthanasia into a positive sentiment shared by many participants:

> After the euthanasia of a couple's cat, the wife tearfully remarks, "You must hate this part of your job." The veterinarian thoughtfully responds, "You know, it is really a blessing to be able to end [the] suffering of animals and to help people say good-bye to their pets. I am fortunate to be able to do this for my patients. We went through heart failure with my granddad, and it was a horrible way to go. Really, [euthanasia] can be a special time for me, because I get to see how much people love their animals."

The tight emotion work of veterinarians helped clients resolve their guilt and reconstruct their identity as good pet owners who, by choosing euthanasia for their animal, made a kind, loving decision. Veterinarians reassured clients: "You gave her a wonderful life, and few people would be willing to go through all you did for her right up to the end. It was the best gift you could give her."

Managing Grief: Veterinarians' Use of Tight and Loose Emotion Management

When managing owners' grief in the negotiation phase, participants had goals similar to those for managing guilt; they strive to control clients' emotions so they can make rational, timely choices. Conversely, after clients make the difficult decision to euthanize their companion animals, clients are no longer expected to suppress, rationalize, or disregard their grief. Clients are allowed to express a wide range of emotions associated with grief (with the exception of guilt), from joy or happiness—imagining good times with their companions—to relief, anxiety, sadness, anger, and nonchalance. Thus, veterinarians managed pet owners' grief after the negotiation phase far more loosely than they did before the decision to euthanize. In contrast to the tight management of guilt, participants engaged in both tight and loose management of their clients' grief.

During negotiations, veterinarians tightly shape the definition of the decision-making process as a nonemotional, rational situation. When clients express grief-related emotions at this time, veterinarians strongly discourage them by ignoring and avoiding the emotion. For example, this veterinarian briefly acknowledged her client's emotional expression but then disregarded it and encouraged him to concentrate on the medical problem at hand: "I know that this is upsetting for you, but now is not the time to get upset. We need to focus. We have to think about making the best decision we can for Dolce. We either need to go ahead with the surgery or decide it is time to stop." Another veterinarian avoided his client's emotional expression by ending the interaction: "I can see that you need some time to collect yourself and think about this decision. Feel free to use the phone if you need to discuss things with your son. Dial this number when you are ready or if you have any questions."

Participants often described the process of ignoring, disregarding, and avoiding clients' grief as *medicalizing* their interactions with clients, as Dr. Hill explained:

> The intense philosophical questions [of euthanasia] are naturally emotion laden, but we try to get the owners to calm down and focus so they make the most informed decision. Sometimes they are so distraught, . . . you have to go over it as rationally and calmly as you can—over and over until their emotions are no longer in the way of

the medical facts. You just have to help them push through their emotions until they understand what is at stake for their animal.

Although it was difficult for participants to disregard their clients' grief, they often did so out of concern for their patients, as Dr. Arford explained: "It is no good [for the patient] to try and sugarcoat it and be all touchy-feely [and] stepping around the truth for the owners. . . . Based on your medical knowledge, if you think the animal is suffering, you sometimes have to use the word *suffering* and not sugarcoat it because you think it might hurt some feelings."

In line with the belief that emotions interfere with good decision making, medicalizing the discussion tightly shapes the impression of the veterinarian as an impartial, rational, expert advisor whose advice is based on science and rationality rather than feelings and attachment. The veterinarian works to maintain a typical veterinary consultation: formal, professional, and lacking intimacy. This atmosphere is aided by using sterile examination rooms in which veterinarians wear white medical coats with stethoscopes and present themselves as the medical model of detached concern maintaining a professional distance.[35] Aside from an occasional handshake, veterinarians carefully avoid touching clients. Conversations are generally limited to the animal's current medical condition and discussions instrumental in obtaining a diagnosis. When the content is considered irrelevant, veterinarians are quick to redirect the conversation by interrupting with questions.

Once a client had decided on euthanasia, participants reacted a great deal differently to clients' grief than they did during the negotiation phase. A noticeable change occurred in the demeanor of many veterinarians. No longer concerned with the potential influence of emotions on the outcome of negotiations, veterinarians acknowledge grief and that coming to such a decision is often agonizing. Dr. Miller described how she transitioned into what many participants described as euthanasia mode:

> I make this conscious transition. . . . I may go from a very business-like or intellectual or even slightly argumentative [position]. If I feel that they are giving me shit and they're not really listening to me, . . . I'm going to be pushing for my point just a little. But once they've made that decision and it's clear, then I'm transitioning to the totally supportive, totally compassionate person . . . to try and help them out emotionally [and] to let them know it is okay to let their feelings out.

Participants often had to suppress their own anger, sadness, and disappointment to transition into euthanasia mode. Although most veterinarians considered patient advocacy an important part of their job, they thought their job also included helping clients deal with the death of their animal or, at least, helping them feel "their grief is appreciated and appropriate." No longer concerned with negotiating possible outcomes for patients, most participants' goals changed to "providing a safe space to grieve for animals" that has "an atmosphere conducive to the expression of emotion."

To achieve this new goal, veterinarians used a variety of emotion-management techniques concurrently and consecutively (see Table 3.1). For example, oral expressions of sympathy and empathy often accompanied non-oral behavior such as a comforting touch. Some participants relied heavily on listening when they were not confident in their ability to offer effective counsel to grieving clients. Of course, a veterinarian's choice of strategy is shaped by the type of relationship between client and veterinarian, the perceived personality of the client, and the disposition of the veterinarian. Strategies such as a comforting touch, for example, might seem inappropriate if the owner is standoffish or unresponsive to such gestures. Not surprisingly, veterinarians used physical strategies such as a hug more frequently with clients with whom they had established some rapport.

After the decision to euthanize has been made, veterinarians expect (and consider warrantable) pet owners to express grief over the loss of their animal. Loose emotion work encouraged clients to see the veterinary office as a space where they could let their feelings out and in which it was safe to express deep sadness over the loss of an animal. However, in the negotiation phase, tight emotion work required pet owners to strictly conform to only one context—a context inconsistent with emotionality. In other words, participants tightly suppressed clients' grief to achieve instrumental goals during negotiations, but they also achieved expressive goals by allowing a cathartic release of emotions. Thus, in the negotiating phase, veterinarians asserted significant authority in shaping sentiments and defining the situation, but after the death of the animal, they allowed clients greater freedom in expressing their feelings.

Creating Affection in a Professional Setting

Upon the death of their animal, clients had the freedom to define the situation in any way they chose. Some pet owners freely expressed their emotions with little prompting from the veterinarian. Yet other pet owners, although feeling intense grief, were reluctant to express it. The display of intimate emotions disrupts the norms of emotional expression between strangers in a professional environment.[36] Erving Goffman suggests that people tend to

TABLE 3.1   STRATEGIES FOR LOOSELY MANAGING CLIENT GRIEF AFTER THE DECISION TO EUTHANIZE

Strategy	Definition	Examples/Explanations
Catharsis	Coaxing the client to express/talk about felt emotions.	"If you need to talk about anything, I am here for you. Would you like me to stay with you?"
Empathy	Understanding/identification with the client's experience by proclamation of similar emotions.	"I lost my cat of nine years to the same kind of cancer just last year. It was a terrible process. I understand exactly what you are feeling right now."
Sympathy	Stating or expressing an emotion for the owner (feeling for the owner).	"It looks like this was very painful for you. You obviously care deeply for Scratchers. It was a terrible accident."
Reassurance	Verbally instilling confidence in the owner (that his or her grief is normal and legitimate).	"I can see that you really loved him, and it is natural to cry and grieve when we experience loss. Many people grieve for their pets. They are important parts of our families."
Redirection	Encouraging the owner to focus on positive memories of the pet rather than on the pet's death.	"I ask the owner, 'Have you had [the pet] since [the animal was] a kitten or a puppy?' And then I try to get [the owner] to think of those moments—the good times—when [the animal] wasn't sick."
Comforting touch	Putting a hand on the owner's body (shoulder or hand) or offering a hug. Touching the animal may also be included.	"If you are not the kind of person who feels comfortable touching the person, then make sure you touch or pet the animal in the process . . . to let the [owner] know that you care."
Body language/gestures	Using body language or gestures to provide emotional support or convey sympathy.	"I just try to look sympathetic and convey through body language that I'm sorry. Taking the time to give [the owner] a Kleenex is a form of communication. You are bonding with [the person] through interaction without words."
Listening	Listening attentively to clients' stories about their animals or whatever they choose to talk about.	"I think just being there makes [the owner] feel better to some extent. Even though I am really busy, I try to let [the owner] talk. It seems like the right thing to do. There is only so much you can say to comfort a person. You don't really know [the person], but you can listen. . . . That is a gift too."

Note: Several strategies (catharsis, empathy, sympathy, and reassurance) mirror those operationalized by DeCoster (1997).

align their emotions according to the norms of expression expected in social settings (the emotional order), and when someone violates the norms people are generally upset and embarrassed.[37]

The emotion work of the veterinarian helps repair the interactional breakdowns during veterinarian-client interactions.[38] Under ordinary circumstances, the veterinarian-client encounter is a sterile, formal professional one between relative strangers, noticeably lacking in emotional intimacy. During the negotiation phases I observed, when clients' emotions were not wanted, the veterinarian's tight emotion management helped restore the emotional order by enforcing the norms of emotional expression typically expected in professional-client relationships. Veterinarians needed to make only a small effort to help owners pull themselves together because, as Goffman notes, people are dedicated to maintaining the social order.[39] Nevertheless, for some clients, the exceptional circumstances of contemplating the death of their pet hindered their ability to sustain desired impressions and they required considerable emotion management to conform to the veterinarian's demands.

After the negotiation phase, the veterinarian's loose emotion work resolved awkward interactions with emotional clients. In these situations the veterinarian changed the norms of expression for the veterinarian-client relationship. In other words, through loose emotion work, veterinarians encouraged clients to see their office as a safe space where they could express grief and feel comfortable enough to freely let their feelings out. For example, in Table 3.1 a veterinarian says, "Taking the time to give [the owner] a Kleenex is a form of communication." Although this may not be the veterinarian's exact intention, something as simple as placing a box of tissues in front of a client communicates that tears are acceptable under these circumstances. Moreover, by encouraging clients to bring friends or family members to support them and drive them home, participants let the client know from the start that emotional expression was typical, acceptable, and expected.

To create an environment conducive to the expression of emotions, the formality of the traditional doctor-client relationship—relied on in almost every other veterinary encounter—must be broken down during euthanasia encounters. Participants let pet owners know that euthanasia was a more informal occasion by making special exceptions to formal rules:

> With euthanasia I like to be more flexible, so if it is decided that they are going to euthanize, they may want to visit and stay with their animals and say good-bye [but their animals are in the intensive care unit] and it isn't visiting hours, and they may be in the way, but I will let them do it anyway. . . . I always want to have some level

of compassion, but with euthanasia I am more willing to bend over backwards and break rules.

Although it is not usual, veterinarians sometimes cry, expressing sympathy or empathy for their clients: "Probably for the first five years I was in practice there was hardly a euthanasia I did with an owner present that I didn't cry. I still often cry with the owners." Dr. Hill described her transition once her clients have decided on euthanasia:

> You move out of those medical modes into the compassionate eutha-
> nasia mode. It brings in all of that emotion, like the compassion and
> feelings. With men, I try to—I don't force anything on them, but I
> try to present it so it's okay for you to feel emotional. So you may have
> used all of your rational facilities to make the decisions to euthanize,
> but now we're letting that go. . . . I make that transition whether they
> have made it or not—not that I'm going to force them to be like, you
> have to deal with your feelings, but I make this conscious transition
> in terms of my demeanor.

Thus, changes in the veterinarian's attitude coupled with the loose emotion-management strategies described earlier change the typical emotional order of veterinarian-client interactions and allow the client to feel comfortable showing emotions.

The incorporation of intimacy between relative strangers into an environment that is, under ordinary circumstances, a sterile, formal professional

Despite the veterinarian's permission to express emotions during eutha-nasia encounters, clients were often uncomfortable and even embarrassed when expressing their grief. Tearful pet owners frequently dismissed their expressions of grief as "stupid," "crazy," or "ridiculous" and apologized for their behavior with disparaging remarks such as "This is so embarrassing. I can't believe I am crying like this." Veterinarians helped their clients salvage their "spoiled identity"[40] by normalizing almost any emotional or physical reaction of their client to the death of their companion animal. For example, veterinarians normalized crying by telling owners, "Everybody does it," or "Oh, this is nothing. We see a lot worse every day." Participants helped embarrassed clients save face[41] by reassuring them their behavior was permit-ted and understandable given their significant loss: "That's okay; it's normal you should be upset. This is your dog; this is your baby. You've had her for this long."

The incorporation of intimacy between relative strangers into an envi-ronment that is, under ordinary circumstances, a sterile, formal professional one is frequent. In their research, Stanford Gregory and Stephen Keto found that veterinarians and their clients express emotions not usually allowed in doctor-patient encounters.[42] During euthanasia situations owners and veterinarians depart from everyday rules of social interactions regulating the outward expression of emotion in front of nonintimates, as described by this veterinarian: "Euthanasia is a very personal and private thing, and here you are sharing it with someone who is essentially a stranger. You know it is the sort of thing where people will fall apart. People . . . don't want to be seen crying, and here they are crying, and they let you see it so they really have opened themselves up to you and made themselves vulnerable."

Euthanasia and Veterinarian-Client Interaction: A Strange Intimacy

Through the use of expressive emotion-management strategies, veterinarians allow, encourage, or at least accept the expression of intimate emotions during euthanasia. Grief, most often expressed through crying, is often accompanied by other intimate interactions, such as touching, hugging, and sharing personal information with gradually increasing ease. Some clients can surprise even the most experienced veterinarians in their eventual willingness to display intimate feelings, weep openly, and reveal details of their lives to people who are basically strangers. For example, these two veterinarians described their experiences with the level of intimacy that clients share during euthanasia:

When they say things during a euthanasia, the kind of stuff they say is a lot more intimate in a way. The way they will tell them they love them is more—more serious, and they tell them all the things they are going to miss about their animal, like going to the park and playing with the Frisbee. The animal doesn't understand them, so when they talk to the animal, what happens is that they are actually sharing these very personal, private thoughts out loud with me.

I had a guy once whose wife was not present when we euthanized the dog, but the two of them had brought the dog in. This relationship was a very surface one, as I had not known them before and only just admitted their dog into the emergency room. . . . I had just euthanized the dog and was kind of giving him a minute to collect himself, and he says to me, "You know, I loved that dog more than my wife." I mean, people just say pretty personal things like that.

As the next two quotations from participants show, veterinarians were sometimes troubled by the personal information that clients revealed:

> People share some unbelievable personal information. . . . [A] lot of people have shared information with me that I am not comfortable with, like very personal illnesses, personal problems with other family members—a lot of what's going on in their life. It's strange. . . . They decide it's okay to do things that they otherwise wouldn't. I don't know why that is. . . . Several times I've sat with people for half an hour, forty-five minutes, where they just talk—sometimes about their pet, sometimes about themselves, sometimes about absolutely nothing at all.

> They might tell me about their own health problems, like right before or right after. . . . Afterwards they want to talk to you and just talk about weird things, personal things. They talk about everything. I have heard about divorces and all kinds of stuff. It is a bit awkward. . . . It is awkward when they share things not related to their pet. They see you as a person to talk to so they do, and they are really emotional so they talk about everything without filter.

Some clients would want to talk with the veterinarians for hours, such that the veterinarian had to end the interaction. Owners have even been known to ask the veterinarian for their home or cellular phone number. Although some veterinarians have given out their private numbers, most offer clients the number of grief hotlines or recommend a local grief counselor or pet support group. While veterinarians want owners to feel comfortable with their expressions of emotionality, they sometimes had to set limits.

From the perspective of the veterinarian, being confronted with the emotion of a stranger or nonintimate can make them uncomfortable, ill at ease, or even embarrassed. The majority of participants experienced the intimacy during euthanasia as at least mildly uncomfortable, if not downright strange. On the one hand, participants made it clear that owners' emotional displays during euthanasia were, given the circumstances, acceptable and legitimate. On the other hand, they also admitted to varying degrees that the intimacy between strangers could be an odd situation. One veterinarian summed it up this way: "Although we try to make it seem normal, I think a lot of people are aware that it's kind of weird to want a hug from somebody they don't know." Yet veterinarians consistently offer varying levels of social and emotional support.[43]

Some participants reconciled their discomfort by resigning themselves to a certain amount of uneasiness during euthanasia for the benefit of the pet owner:

> I have had owners give me hugs, and I have even had kisses—on the cheek, but I have had kisses. They kind of creep me out. [*Laughs.*] Strangers literally put their lips on my face. It is kind of scary. They will want a hug, and so I will give them a hug. . . . It kind of hurts [*laughs*], but whatever. It's just awkward to get a hug from someone that you don't even know. You've only seen their animal for the ten minutes that you saw them—like, it's just a little weird. . . . There are a lot of people that I've known for a long time that I've never hugged, and they are friends. So I've never hugged certain friends, let alone [initiated a hug with] someone that I just met.

Moreover, rejecting a pet owner's request for counsel or a hug might disrupt the interaction and make the veterinarian feel worse: "I am not a huggy or touchy person, but if they go to hug me, I will go along with it. It is not the time to be like, 'Wow, buddy!' It would be more awkward to *not* hug them. . . . You don't want any client to feel weird and awkward and embarrassed that they want to shake your hand or hug you and you pushed them away on top of they just euthanized their pet." Although difficult at times, most participants attempted to hide their discomfort from the owners to minimize disruption.

Participants carefully monitored their expression of emotions even with clients for whom sympathy and compassion were not easy to muster. As illustrated in Chapter 2, veterinarians do emotional labor by carefully monitoring their expressions of emotions during euthanasia performances to create a good last memory of their pet for their clients.[44] I argue, and Goffman might agree, that veterinarians tend to have excellent dramaturgical discipline because they are able to maintain a consistent performance in the face of challenges.[45] As mentioned previously, participants validated euthanasia choices even when they were upset or angered with clients, supporting even those seen as not worthy of sympathy and compassion. Similar to the experience of prison officers and criminal justice workers, veterinarians sometimes had trouble managing their anger and instead displaying compassion and sympathy for individuals perceived as unworthy of such emotions.[46] Yet participants often suppressed their own anger, sadness, and disappointment to transition into euthanasia mode.

Most participants felt obligated at some point in their career to listen to the adventures of a client's pet for an hour or hug a stranger because the context of euthanasia warranted their inconvenience or discomfort. Sometimes the context of euthanasia provides enough rationale for intimacy with a stranger that it renders the intimacy benign: "Tons of people hug us, tons of people. With euthanasia you almost expect them to hug you. It doesn't bother me because I know that it is a totally different type of contact. We all know that it is related to euthanasia, so it really doesn't make us uncomfortable." Thus, when veterinarians feel ill at ease because owners express emotions, share personal details regarding their life, and seek physical contact, they think of the intimacy as legitimate or acceptable because it is within the exceptional and temporary context of euthanasia.

Participants defining their clients as strangers made the intimacy feel strange or uncomfortable; however, feeling connected to the owner alleviated some of the awkwardness. For example, Dr. Miller explained how her discomfort with hugging clients was lessened when she had developed a special connection: "With those people I get to know more I would reciprocate [the hug] and not think about it versus reciprocating and thinking how uncomfortable it is with more of a stranger and be really glad when it is over." For some veterinarians, like Dr. Jones, this strategy worked well because they were able to easily redefine the client's status from stranger to familiar:

> There are some people [clients] who come in and sit with their animal at every visiting hour and beg you to let them stay longer. . . . Most are about a week, I would say, but I mean, it is contact every single day—two to three times a day or at least twice per day contact. You are their connection to their pet when the pet is in the hospital. It can be an intense time. . . . You can really get to know an owner when they are around like that.

This veterinarian could feel more at ease with intimacy because she was able to reframe the relationship. However, this strategy did not work as well for other veterinarians, such as Dr. Arford, who more narrowly defined familiarity:

> We don't tend to develop long-term relationships with clients just 'cause of the nature of our service [emergency medicine]. You are a stranger to them really. You sort of bond over the few days or weeks that the patient is in the hospital, and there is a level of trust, and they trust you and your competency and medical judgment, but they are still strangers. . . . I don't think that I have established relationships

with clients; . . . probably most vets who do that are people who have [clients] that they have seen those animals from a puppy to an older pet. . . . I can imagine it would be different if I had more of a relationship with the family or the people.

Notice that Dr. Jones and Dr. Arford are both emergency veterinarians, work in the same department, and describe similar experiences with clients, but Dr. Arford views her clients almost exclusively as strangers and continues to have difficulties with intimacy. Nonstranger relationships are generally determined by how much time the veterinarian spends with clients, the veterinarian's identification with the client or the animal, or the intensity of the interaction for the veterinarian (e.g., dramatic critical cases). Compared to participants with attitudes similar to Dr. Arford's, participants like Dr. Jones reported little strange intimacy because, for them, many of their clients were not defined as strangers.

For a few veterinarians the strange intimacy of euthanasia is rarely problematic—regardless of their relationship with owners—because the intimacy informs their professional identity. For these veterinarians the physical contact and intimacy with owners during euthanasia enhances their identity as a veterinarian who is kind and compassionate. Similar to Dr. Ferguson, several participants suggested that helping grieving clients with their emotions was part of what attracted them to the profession in the first place:

When I was in college, I always said that I was going to go into human medicine. And . . . probably . . . half the reason I went into veterinary medicine—not human medicine—is because my veterinarian was a much more emotional person. When my horse was sick, he would give me a hug, but my own family doctor probably would not give me a hug if he were telling me that Mom had just passed away. Human doctors are more—in my experience—much more emotionally distant and [have a] rigid bedside manner that I have never experienced with veterinarians. Veterinarians have always seemed more emotional or comfortable people.

Compared to some of his colleagues, Dr. Black took pride in having more compassion and willingness to allow intimacy into euthanasia encounters:

When owners tell you they had their other dog put down with another vet who was just much colder and they appreciate your compassion, that is great. What you did for them was nicer and made it easier for them than what they have had in the past. . . . It is the compassion and the little things like a hug or going slow and taking the time to listen to them and saying nice things. . . . I don't mind it, but I think that some vets do. Some people are not like that. Some veterinarians I won't say are not capable, but that is just not something that they are wired to do. For me, compassion is a very important part of being a vet.

Having empathy and, more importantly, the ability to convey it to clients during the stressful time of pet loss is a key part of these veterinarians' definition of what it means to be a good veterinarian.

Regardless of their comfort level, participants' actions outlined in this chapter demonstrate that veterinarians are rethinking old notions of professional responsibility to include offering comfort and counsel to clients whose animals they euthanize. Even those participants for whom intimacy is less easily negotiated still reported feeling responsible to their clients when it came to the death of their patients. For example, Dr. Green nicely articulated her sense of responsibility when it comes to euthanasia:

Most of what we do in euthanasia with owners is not technically a part of our job as veterinarians. I know this stuff is above and beyond, but I feel like that *is* my job. It's like that is our part as part funeral director. It's not like we're just doctors. We're part healer, part grief counselor, part funeral director, so of course we have that feeling that [it] is our responsibility to make euthanasia go well for the animal and the owner.

Most participants believed that it is the responsibility of veterinarians to validate and legitimate owners' grief over their animal. They often reported a duty to be there for owners, especially given that others in society may not understand their grief or demonstrate sufficient sympathy toward their loss. For some veterinarians the comfort they offered clients felt natural because they were extremely empathetic to animals and the bonds people share with them, yet for other veterinarians the bonds they felt toward animals offered them little help when it came to comforting clients.

During my research it became clear to me that small-animal veterinarians consider the business of veterinary service to include maintaining the health and well-being of animals *and* attending to the emotional needs of their clients. Participants provided literature on pet loss and recommended books to their clients. Across the country, veterinarians are joining with mental health professionals to offer referrals to local therapists specializing in pet loss, and some even employ full-time counselors to assist grieving pet owners.[47] Some clinics sponsor regular support-group sessions. Recall from Chapter 2 that veterinarians sell urns, caskets, jewelry, and other products designed for memorializing deceased pets. They increasingly invest in designer spaces for euthanasia known as meditation, comfort, or grieving rooms with soothing wall colors, comfortable seating, and low lighting. Although helping owners through the death of their animals may be a big practice builder, these acts show a growing commitment by the veterinary profession to recognize the intense grief, pain, and sorrow resulting from the death of a pet.

Euthanasia and Veterinarian-Client Interaction: A Unique Socioemotional Exchange

The affective role veterinarians assume in comforting bereaved pet owners initiates an unexpected response. Compared to times when veterinarians cure or restore health to the animal, clients are far *more* likely to offer their veterinarians gratitude for ending the lives of companion animals. Dr. Black explained the curious gratitude response:

> People love you if you kill their animal right. If you save an animal, they might be like, "Oh, thanks," and then they leave. The people whose animals you euthanize and show them compassion and you are nice to them, they love it. I have more letters from people whose animals I have killed compared to animals that I have saved. There are people who are very grateful when you help their animal, but when you euthanize an animal, they are *much more* grateful and *much more* thankful.

Participants received four to five times the cards or gifts from clients after euthanasia than from other veterinary consultation. Most cards, letters, photographs, gift certificates, gourmet food, flowers, gift baskets, and monetary donations to special hospital funds come from clients after the death of their animal. Some clients go to similar lengths to show gratitude for the veterinarian's life-saving efforts but most do not, and the difference between the latter and euthanasia clients is striking. Indeed, not long into their internships the desks of novice interns quickly filled with displays of euthanasia-related gratitude, and seasoned participants estimated they have received several hundred such gifts over the course of their careers. Although appreciative of their clients' gestures, veterinarians are often baffled by the level of gratitude for what they see as essentially an unsuccessful service—ending with the death of the pet.

That veterinarians are far more likely to receive gratitude for euthanasia compared to times when they restored the animal's health is curious. This gratitude pattern stands in sharp contrast to the gratitude pattern experienced by Lois's rescue workers.[48] Rescue workers experienced a complete opposite response from family members when their loved one died. When victims were saved gratitude was lavished on the workers, yet when death occurred, family members rarely offered gratitude for the service provided them. Lois speculates that, when the victim died, family members did not feel obligated to provide gratitude because "socioemotional norms dictated that the families' emotional grief and bad fortune far outweighed the emotional support the rescuers had provided during the mission."[49] By comparison, why did clients send so many more gestures of gratitude when their companion animals died than when the veterinarian saved the animal? Shouldn't pet owners' bad fortune—loss of a pet—also outweigh the emotional support they were provided?

Candace Clark's notion of the "socioemotional economy"[50] coupled with Arnold Arluke and Clinton Sanders's concept of a "sociozoologic scale"[51] help answer these questions. Clark's socioemotional economy suggests that sympathy is an important emotional resource such that when exchanged between people they "limit sympathy depending on what they know, think they know, or suspect about a person's social value. Social value entitles a person to sympathy margins. The greater one's social value the wider and deeper the margins others create for him or her."[52] At the same time, societal value is determined by one's position along the sociozoologic scale. As a person's position changes over time, society may worship, protect, segregate, or seek to destroy the person. Most humans are on top at any given time, and the closer an animal is to humans' position, the less society will tolerate, ignore, or condone their mistreatment. The higher an animal's position on the sociozoologic scale, the more its death is seen as worthy of human grief and the sympathy of others.

Dogs and cats sit much higher on the sociozoologic scale compared to other animals such as mice and poultry, and those who cherish their canine or feline companions often do not understand the grief felt by mice or chicken enthusiasts over the loss of such animals. Recall the cases of the euthanasia of the chicken and the mouse from the Introduction. Although many of us try to keep mice out of our homes—exterminating them as pests—others cherish their companionship and consult veterinarians to ensure their health and well-being. Nevertheless, the owner's grief at the loss of his beloved Sam and the staff's inability to understand his reaction to the mouse's death reflects the logic of the sociozoologic scale. In other words, despite some people's attraction and dedication to a mouse or chicken, the sociozoologic scale suggests that most people in society will relate to their death in much the same way the young veterinarian did of his patient: "It's no big deal—it's *just* a chicken."

Grief over the death of a companion animal is socially less legitimate than grief over the loss of a spouse, child, or parent because of their different positions on the sociozoologic scale. When a human family member dies most people are surrounded by nurturing friends and family, but they rarely receive the same attention when their companion animal dies. Despite some pet owners experiencing greater bonds with animals than they do with humans,[53] scholars note a broad societal tendency to trivialize grief over the loss of an animal companion.[54] Kenneth Doka coined the term "disenfranchised grief" to describe situations in which someone experiences a significant loss but is denied the "right to grieve" because the bereavement is not openly acknowledged, socially validated, or publicly observed.[55] When people grieve for the loss of their pets, their grief may be exacerbated by the social negation of their loss.[56] One survey of pet owners found that more than 50 percent of respondents believed that society did not view the death of a pet as a loss worthy of grief.[57]

In light of the often documented ambiguity inherent in human-animal relationships discussed in the Introduction,[58] some simply do not understand pet owners' intense feelings of grief over the death of their companion animal of whatever species. Although some friends and family may want to comfort loved ones after the death of a beloved animal, they may not fully understand or appreciate the loss. For example, the well-intended suggestion, "You might feel better if you just go get another dog," can seem to some pet owners the same as if someone were to say to a grieving widower, "Don't worry; you can easily get a new wife." Other acquaintances, colleagues, and friends may even believe that grieving for animals is silly or overly sentimental and respond to the loss with an insensitive remark, such as "It's *only* a cat. What's the big deal?"

According to the sociozoologic scale, people accord humans a higher status than to nonhuman animals. And according to the socioemotional economy, differing sympathy reactions reflect the narrow sympathy margins for the loss of those deemed less worthy. By combining the sociozoologic scale and the socioemotional economy, we see that pet owners are not owed the same kind of sympathy reserved for a death in the family because society creates restricted sympathy margins for the loss of nonhuman animals. Yet as we have seen in this chapter, veterinarians encourage clients to see the veterinary office as a safe place to express deep sadness over the loss of companion animals. This is the reason that pet owners feel obligated to provide gratitude: because reciprocity norms dictate that they are not owed the sympathy and emotional support they received from veterinarians for their loss.

While veterinarians are often baffled by the level of gratitude they receive for euthanasia, evidence suggests that clients respond, at least in part, to the affective role veterinarians assume in validating grief over the death of animals. Hochschild, in her concept of economy of gratitude, argues that people offer each other gratitude only when their behavior is thought to go above and beyond what is expected.[59] Clients, according to economy of gratitude, feel obligated to respond to euthanasia with gratitude because they believe they are getting something extra that is not paid for in the typical fee-for-service exchange. In the typical veterinary consultation, no extra gratitude is deemed necessary because veterinarians receive monetary fees in equal exchange for services they provide the client. However, when it comes to euthanasia, clients are never billed for the extras such as the time veterinarians spend providing emotional support. When veterinarians receive many more gestures of gratitude related to euthanasia compared to other services, this seemingly paradoxical response of pet owners is a logical, appropriate reaction to a valuable service—veterinary emotion work.

In further support of these interpretations, the content of euthanasia-related cards and letters sent by clients demonstrates that clients recognize and appreciate the emotion work of their veterinarians. For example, clients wrote, "Thank you for helping us through such a tough time," "Thank you for your kindness, compassion, and understanding," and "Thank you for helping us come to such a difficult decision." Clients often mentioned specific emotion-management strategies such as listening and "being there" for the client. Pet owners often wrote that they appreciated the veterinarian's validation of their grief: "You really get my loss in a way that other people who don't have pets just can't understand—that bond we have with our animals." In addition to grief, clients also frequently mentioned the veterinarian's efforts to help them resolve feelings of guilt: "I just had so much guilt over not catching his cancer earlier, but you helped me know how difficult it is to see when some animals are sick because they are stubborn or brave like Dawson. You helped me to finally say good-bye to my beloved friend."

As we have seen, the emotion-laden encounters between veterinarians and bereaved pet owners provide a rich context for examining professionals' management of the emotions of clients in the workplace. To accomplish their task, veterinarians assuage emotions to facilitate timely, rational decisions, but they also create space for the expression of intimate feelings between strangers in a professional setting. Veterinarians express empathy and sympathy—they listen to owners, reassure them, offer a comforting touch on the arm or stroke the animal's fur, and may even hug the owners. Denying the legitimacy of guilt, veterinarians reassure pet owners that they made a loving decision in the best interest of the animal. Grief over the death of an animal companion is reinforced as normal and appropriate given the situation and indicative of the behavior of good and loving pet owners.

My research for this book did not explore the pet owner's perspective, but many veterinarians strongly argued that dealing with client emotions is essential to client satisfaction and building long-term relationships with clients. Dr. Mulford hypothesized that creating a safe space for grieving clients strengthens veterinarian-client relationships:

> I find that, if anything, you know they appreciate that you are a professional, but they also appreciate that you empathize because we all—as pet owners—get attitude from people: "Oh, it's just a dog" or "Oh, it's just a cat." You know the flippancy of how pets are considered in the press or in the media or society or whatever, and I think people really appreciate knowing that, while you are a professional, you are also empathetic. . . . You understand their bond.

Perhaps, as Dr. Mulford suggested, pet owners appreciate veterinarians' creation of rituals for the death of animals (as described in Chapter 2) and are grateful for the emotional support and validation of their loss. And as we have seen, veterinarians must manage their clients' grief within a cultural context that often fails to provide pet owners with sufficient emotional support for the loss of a beloved animal companion. Though memorial gardens and pet cemeteries have long existed to entomb the remains of companion animals, rituals for the public expression of grief over the death of animals are still rare.[60]

Although evidence from this study suggests that clients respond, at least in part, to the affective role veterinarians assume in validating grief over a pet's death, more research is needed on clients' perspective. This research has important implications for veterinary practitioners because it illuminates an often veiled or ignored aspect of the profession. Though managing clients' emotions is not generally considered an official aspect of a veterinarian's job description, my research suggests that small-animal veterinarians are doing emotion work. Veterinarians believe they provide important emotional support to clients,[61] and pet owners thank their veterinarians specifically for providing them comfort and counsel. Although some veterinarians consider such emotion work outside their domain of knowledge, experience, and responsibility, my research reveals that many veterinarians are rethinking old notions of professional responsibility to include managing the emotions of clients whose animals they euthanize.

4

Learning to Euthanize

Death and the Novice Veterinarian

Similar to any novice to an unknown subculture, I entered the daily lives of veterinarians with only anticipations of what I might experience and how I might think, feel, and behave. First and foremost, I had to adjust to sights and smells that initially made me woozy. During the early stages of my fieldwork, I found it especially difficult to hide my physical discomfort with nauseating puss-filled wounds and the body storage and cremation areas. However, after a few solid weeks of transporting dead animals' remains, I became so accustomed to them that I could easily eat food in the same room with them. Moreover, the previously overwhelming sights and smells no longer fazed me as I became caught up in the drama of medical mysteries, and I began to watch in curious amazement as the veterinarians around me dealt with the various colors and textures seeping from open wounds.

Given that I had never spent much time in the backrooms of a busy animal hospital, I had to get used to the flurry of activity and commotion. When it came to interacting with animal patients, I quickly learned of the potential hazards and how to avoid dangerous mishaps. I learned my first lesson when a young, approximately seventy-pound Alaskan malamute lunged at me while the veterinarian tested his reflexes. Luckily, it was only a warning to back off; however, his angry growl and serious intent to perhaps eat my face off did make me question my commitment to the research. In any event, I grew quite comfortable around patients, even those who were not altogether pleased by their trip to see the veterinarian. Over time, I adjusted to the hustle and bustle of a busy emergency hospital and began to gather information that both confirmed and challenged my initial beliefs.

In the beginning many of my expectations about the job were challenged. For example, I was amazed by the number of stressed-out clients who brought healthy animals to the hospital during emergency hours for minor or imagined conditions. At the same time, other, dispassionate clients, either unconcerned about the severity of their animal's condition or unaware of it, brought them to the hospital days or weeks too late. Many pets were killed because owners were ignorant of the animal's basic needs, preventive medicine, or proper care. Some simply did not understand the time and financial commitment that comes with owning a pet.

As an academic interested in human-animal relationships, I was well-read on the ambiguous and contradictory attitudes of people toward nonhuman animals; however, I was often taken aback by the reality. Some people generously paid for the medical care of injured wildlife or stray animals found in their neighborhood, while other people tried to poison their neighbors' animals for trespassing onto their property. One case I will not soon forget involved an elderly man who, while out walking his dog, was pushed to the ground while a stranger nearly kicked his dog to death. Another client wanted to euthanize her cat because she had family members coming into town who were allergic to cats. She said she was not much of an animal person and the cat whined too much anyway. At the same time, I could tell that many participants took pleasure in their work, in part because they enjoyed being around animals and often had strong bonds with their own companion animals.

As a novice to the world of veterinarians, my initial expectations about how I might feel were seriously tested. First, I have been told I am much more of a rational person than an especially sensitive one—meaning I am not a stone, but my heartstrings are rarely pulled, so to speak. Although I anticipated seeing animal suffering and watching bereaved clients, I quickly realized that imagining those situations was an entirely different matter to seeing them for myself. My first lesson came in the form of an Irish wolfhound named Murphy brought into the hospital in the wee hours of the morning following Thanksgiving Day. While the family enjoyed their post-turkey naps and television, Murphy snuck into the kitchen to finish off the leftovers on the table. I learned that the stomach of large-breed dogs like Murphy who eat and drink a lot and then roll around playing can twist around itself— potentially a life-threatening situation. It was now several hours since he had first started to show symptoms and he was in critical condition. The surgery would be expensive and was not guaranteed to save his life. Murphy's owners, a local firefighter and second-grade teacher, were clearly distraught over his unexpected condition. It was obvious that they were not wealthy people and were clearly torn about the financial sacrifice they would have to make, but they did not take long to decide to go for the surgery.

Even though I had been on shift since about 6:00 P.M. Thanksgiving Day, I stayed for the surgery and went back and forth updating the clients as instructed by the resident I was shadowing. When the surgeons opened the dog's stomach I was incredulous at the amount of food and water he had consumed. Joking with his owners, I listed some of the contents Murphy had inhaled. Proud of their Irish heritage, the couple explained that Murphy's name comes from a Celtic word meaning "hound of the sea." Because the man sometimes referred to Murphy as Madreen, I asked if that was the Celtic pronunciation. He laughed and explained that *madreen* was a Celtic word meaning "little puppy" but also a slang term for "tramp." Mistaking his meaning of "tramp" as a term for a promiscuous woman, I made a joke about Murphy being a lady's man. The man laughed and responded in his thick Boston accent, "No, like a bum, 'cause he's always scavenging about for food." I never expected I would get that emotionally invested in a patient, but I also did not anticipate how good it would feel to get to know people who have such intense and special relationships with their animals. In the end, the little tramp pulled through.

The euthanasia procedures I observed were difficult at times but also warm, funny, touching, bittersweet, and sometimes heartbreaking. Pet owners told the most hilarious and heartrending stories as they reflected on their life with the animal: The cat who seemed to never pay her owner any attention but always came to sit with her when she cried. The police dog who took a bullet for his owner and survived ten more years. We heard stories of puppies getting into all sorts of trouble and ruining family treasures. Behavior that clearly annoyed the owners in life seemed cute and endearing after the animal's death. For example, one client's dog, after indulging his taste for decomposition by rolling on a dead badger, ran up to his owner for a big kiss. People loved to talk about the simple pleasure of their animals— a pond, a bird in the window, a treat, a laser pointer, or a nap in the sun. In their storytelling during euthanasia, these pet owners clearly wanted to honor the life of a cherished and loyal four-legged family member: "He taught me to roll with punches, live in the moment, and appreciate all the simple joys of life."

After all these experiences, I often thought, "Are these vets made of steel?" Trained and committed to saving the lives of animals, how do they resist adopting all those animals they would rather not euthanize? Whether a pet faces a life-threatening illness or needs an allergy shot, veterinarians have to be prepared to assume the appropriate mood required by the job. They walk into euthanasia scenes, focus on the animal, stroke their fur, administer the injection, and say to the grieving client, "She's gone." How do they go from that scene directly into the next room and smile at the puppy with a lacerated paw? How do they not cry when someone leans over her dog or cat as he is dying and says, "Yes, yes, darling, you are a good boy. Everything is going to be all right. You are such a brave boy. Mommy loves you." Many times I had to ask myself, "How do they do it?"

The answer is, in part, that in the beginning they did not. There are a lot of veterinarians with one-eyed, three-legged diabetic pets who had been slated for euthanasia. Many veterinarians shed tears during euthanasia procedures, while others tucked themselves away in a bathroom only to emerge red eyed from crying. Before I began my fieldwork among veterinarians, I had read studies showing that the practice of euthanasia was particularly stressful for novice veterinarians.[1] Still, I wanted to learn more details about aspects of euthanasia that novices felt ill prepared or confident to handle as they entered their first year in the real world of veterinary medicine. The techniques veterinarians use to cope with the stressors associated with euthanasia are the focus of Chapter 5, but this chapter is concerned with the experiences of recent veterinary school graduates.

My fieldwork allowed me to shadow an entire cohort of veterinary interns from before their first days in the hospital until their last day of the internship. In the initial interviews, before their internship officially began, I asked interns to recall how and what they had learned about euthanasia in veterinary school from formal classes, laboratories, and clinics, as well as informal interactions with professors and anecdotes shared among students. I asked them what they anticipated the positive and negative aspects of euthanasia would be. I asked them to reflect on their time in veterinary school and evaluate the merits of their euthanasia-related training. I documented their initial fears, anxieties, and concerns in the interviews, and then I remained with them as they grew and matured from apprehensive novices into more seasoned professionals.

I was alongside many of the interns the first time they had to give an owner bad news, negotiate with a client on when to euthanize a pet, and for a few, euthanize their first patient. During their four years of veterinary school, interns had seen enough to know what to expect in broad categories, but they had not spoken at length with clients or been directly confronted with the day-to-day dilemmas inherent in the work routine. For example, veterinary students go through several years of intense training in how to save lives and treat diseases using the best technology available at their institutions;

however, many pet owners are not able or willing to pay for sophisticated diagnostic technology and expensive treatment strategies.

Research indicates that novice physicians often hide uncomfortable feelings behind a cloak of confidence to prove themselves worthy and ready to enter the world of medicine.[2] In contrast, although they did sometimes put on their cloak of confidence when among supervisors, I was surprised at how many concerns and vulnerable emotions the interns shared with me about euthanasia throughout their first year in practice. Perhaps the interns felt more at ease with me because they saw me as a pseudopeer, a humble graduate student sincerely interested in their experiences. Some interns at the beginning expressed few concerns and reported little anxiety, while others were quite open about many concerns and anxieties. By the end of their first year, all the interns had been overwhelmed many times by nuances of the job, ones that they had not anticipated as well as those they knew to expect from their earlier training.

Entering the Internship

Students enter veterinary school focused more on animals than pet owners and generally place low importance on their ability to interact effectively with people.[3] However, by the end of their education—right when they are about to enter the professional workplace—their attitudes toward animals and people usually begin to even out. In the beginning of their internship, the interns I studied were particularly concerned with four elements of client interaction regarding euthanasia: negotiating the decision to euthanize, discussing related financial issues, managing the impression of a good death for owners, and dealing with subsequent client emotions. In addition to these concerns, I asked them to talk about their own feelings and emotions regarding euthanasia.

Negotiating the Decision to Euthanize

As veterinary students, many of the interns were rarely involved in the decision-making process leading up to euthanasia. Although interns could recall witnessing exchanges between clients and clinicians, most rarely communicated directly with pet owners during veterinary school. Regardless of their earlier experiences, it was clear in our initial interviews that this issue concerned them, and several cried just thinking about the challenges they might face. Almost all of the interns expressed concern about potential disagreements they might have with clients' decisions. Many were unsure what they would do if pet owners asked them to do something that challenged their ethical beliefs. Some worried about what might happen when their ethical choices or opinions did not match those of their superiors.

When asked what they thought would be the most challenging aspect of euthanasia, several of the interns thought disagreements with owners would be their number-one concern. One intern anticipated difficult disagreements: "A situation that I haven't really had to come into contact with yet but I know it's going to happen this year is euthanizing pets that could easily be fixed or you know are being euthanized for issues that aren't necessarily . . . behavioral or medically necessary. That is definitely something that is going to be very hard for me." By contrast, the most popular response to the question of what they thought would be the most rewarding aspect of euthanasia—next to the ability to relieve suffering—had to do with the owners "doing the right thing at the right time." As one intern put it, "The most rewarding thing, I guess, will be when they know it's time, they know it's right . . . and you know at the same time, . . . and then you do it, and it goes smoothly, and they are so appreciative—that will be rewarding."

Given their relative lack of clinical knowledge and experience, several were concerned that they might miss something or make a mistake that could end in the death of their patient. Specifically, when it came to euthanasia, their concern was that they might influence an owner to choose euthanasia when it was based on an incorrect diagnosis. Before he began his internship, Dr. Marshall expressed his concerns: "Going home the next day and wondering whether I recommended the right thing or not is going to be hard, especially when what I say leads to the killing of an animal." Like a lot of his peers, Dr. Marshall reiterated these same concerns a few months into the internship:

> Being a new vet that doesn't really have a lot of experience, there's been times in the back of my head where I've thought, "What if we could have done something for this pet? What if somebody else had seen it and said, 'Oh, this is easy; you just give it this and send it home'"? . . . Am I killing something that somebody else could have fixed easily? But that's the hardest part that goes through the back of your head—that maybe there is something, and you're missing it, and the animal ends up dead. You can't take back euthanasia. It is final.

Knowing they could be called on to euthanize an animal added to the anxiety novice practitioners often felt regarding their lack of clinical knowledge and experience.

In the beginning of their internships, the thought that they would be euthanizing only animals with serious illnesses comforted many interns;

however, as their first year in practice progressed, they began to run into difficult cases that challenged their idealistic expectations. Not surprisingly, moral conflicts were especially challenging for novice interns. The conflict veterinarians often have between caring for animals and inflicting death is heightened when veterinarians are asked to euthanize animals because of a rationale they believe is illegitimate or morally problematic.[4] Dr. Conrad described her frustration with owners who request euthanasia for reasons she considers merely convenience:

> I will support euthanasia [for] severe aggression . . . but the others, for convenience, like "I am moving" or "He scratches the couch" or "[He] is peeing on the carpet," no. If your landlord doesn't allow pets, find a different apartment. Show some responsibility. This is your pet and your responsibility. I firmly believe that pets are not rights but are luxuries, and if you can't provide for one, then you should not have one. It sounds harsh, but I believe that because I see horrible cases day in and day out where people just want to pass the buck and neglect them. They were great when they were this fuzzy, fun thing, and now that they are vomiting, it is inconvenient. [It] makes me extremely mad when they want euthanasia for stupid reasons.

Interns disliked being confronted with the euthanasia of an animal for trivial reasons, especially those related to the owner seeing the animal as a nuisance or no longer wanting to care for the animal.

Although many interns expected to struggle with aspects of life-and-death decision making, they were surprised how far from clear-cut most decisions seemed. For example, what some clients and colleagues considered legitimate reasons to euthanize seemed more like matters of convenience to the interns. Ideally, many of the interns believed, euthanasia should be a tool for relieving pain and suffering. But they are also called on to euthanize animals when owners cannot afford to treat them or for a rationale not related to illness. Early in their internships, many were upset when approached to euthanize animals with behavior problems such as digging up the yard or loud barking. Because interns saw euthanasia as a tool to end suffering, they also had difficulties with clients who refused to euthanize certain sick animals. In fact, by the end of the internship, several interns suggested that this disagreement was the most upsetting and the most difficult to resolve.

Confronting owners with whom they have disagreements can be a major source of stress for novice practitioners. When asked to euthanize for behavioral problems, for example, many initially felt uncomfortable negotiating alternatives for the patient: "It's hard to just look a client straight in the eye and tell them, 'Look, you're being unethical about things.'" Despite interns anticipating conflict with their clients when negotiating life-and-death issues, they often underestimated how difficult it would be to confront clients themselves:

> It is hard when people bring an animal in to be euthanized that really shouldn't be, because it can get nasty. You can get confrontational. I have had people take their animal and leave. I won't euthanize an animal just because the owner wants me to because it crapped in the house or something like that, but . . . the hardest thing, I think, [is] to have to confront them. We live in a society where people have really different views about animals, and so you are going to get those people who have radically different views than you do. Yeah, they are going to crap on the floor sometimes. Shut up and deal with it. [*Laughs.*] I say that now, but it can be really, really difficult to actually confront these owners. What you are essentially doing in so many words is saying they are morally wrong.

As the interns had anticipated, many struggled with negotiating life-and-death outcomes for their patients and resolving disagreements with clients.

Discussing Financial Issues in Euthanasia

Interns had many concerns about talking with clients over financing an animal's care and what to do when owners cannot or will not pay for care. Several interns reported financial restraints as their number-one concern, as expressed by this intern: "I think the hardest thing about euthanasia is going to be trying to accept the fact that people aren't going to pay for everything that you want to do for the animal in regard to tests and treatment options." At the start of her internship, financial limitations were also Dr. Buford's greatest concern: "It will be euthanizing animals because people don't have enough money to fix them. I'm okay if your pet is very old and very sick and there's really not any other option. I'm comfortable with that. But [I'm not comfortable if] your pet is young and, given $1,000, we could fix it, but you don't have $1,000, so we have to euthanize your pet."

Several participants shared a belief that pet owners who are referred to university hospitals are more financially able to pay for treatment and less negotiation will be needed between the veterinarian and the owner. As a result, interns leaving their internship expect they will have to deal with financial limitations more than they did in their university hospital. A few interns believed the university setting shielded them entirely from purely financially based or unjustified euthanasia: "I think it has been easy for me because I haven't seen any animals I think should not have been euthanized being euthanized. . . . All the cases I have shadowed have been very, very easy: animals that really didn't have any other options. They were in bad shape, and we did all that we could for them." Most of the interns anticipated being asked to euthanize animals for a larger variety of health conditions than they were exposed to at their universities, which in turn would lead to an increase in disagreements with owners.

Many participants believed veterinary school taught them how to diagnose and treat illness without consideration of how finances might influence this process. Thus, many interns felt ill prepared to deal with financial constraints because of a lack of realistic experiences in school, as expressed by this intern: "It would be great if you had all the resources in the world—which is what they teach you in school—if you had everything, what would you do for the animal, hypothetically? But you also have to keep the owners in mind. . . . The owners might not be financially capable of doing everything that they could possibly do for the pet, . . . and then what do you do? They don't teach you that." When clients can't afford the textbook treatment interns learned in school, the interns fear they lack the clinical street smarts, or knowledge of less expensive treatment plans, that could save the patient from euthanasia.

Novices recognize that a veterinarian's ability to accurately estimate the cost of a patient's treatment can have life-and-death consequences for animals in their care. However, as Dr. Arford explained, accurate financial estimates in medicine are inherently difficult:

> We are like mechanics bargaining with people over things, but it is so much worse because medicine is so much more unpredictable. Physiology is way more complicated than a car and exceeds your ability to predict like a mechanic could. Things may go from a $600 estimate to a $3,000 estimate, which is totally realistic, . . . and I bet a lot of medical doctors never really learn how to do this like we have to. It is a necessary skill for us.

Underestimating the cost of treatment can cause mistrust between the veterinarian and the owner as prices gradually rise, while overestimating may lead the owner to choose euthanasia rather than pay to treat. Dr. Turner added, "Underestimating is hard because that ends up bringing out a lot of hard feelings from the owner because then they feel taken advantage of, . . . but I also don't want to discourage people from treating a problem."

Accurate estimates are especially difficult for novice interns who lack the clinical knowledge for precise estimates. Dr. Buford explained how a lack of clinical skills makes it all the more difficult to predict costs:

> It was a learning process of how long do they really need to be in the hospital to treat condition X or Y? What do you really need to do to treat them? Oh, you forgot to estimate for a chest tube or radiograph, things that people tell you that you should do, but maybe when you first initially start out as a doctor you're just not as aware of exactly what you need to do in your workup. You don't have the clinical skills to predict a lot of the costs behind treating different illnesses.

Interns reported significant stress in learning to make estimates and predict costs. Every intern occasionally took heat from hospital administrators who had to fight with angry clients over bloated bills. And every intern experienced stress when he or she believed a high estimate caused the client to choose euthanasia. Naturally, more clinical experience means greater accuracy in predicting outcomes, but it is not a guarantee. Because of the uncertainty inherent in clinical medicine, it is difficult—even for highly experienced veterinarians—to always make accurate estimates.

For many interns, simply talking about funding a patient's care can seem distasteful, and discussion of finances can be especially stressful when the outcome is euthanasia. About midway though her internship, Dr. Clark described her embarrassment and discomfort with discussing the business aspects of veterinary medicine:

> I dread bringing up money when I think it is going to play an important role in the decision to euthanize, because finances are very private—money for a lot of people is a badge of pride. You can see them uncomfortable that they have to make a decision that involves money when it comes to their animals' lives. . . . They don't want to seem like they don't care about their animal. They don't want to seem like they don't have money. And it sucks. It embarrasses me. But it happens a lot that they have to make that decision, and it comes down to money, and that is awkward, and we have to kill their pet because they can't pay.

I was not surprised to hear interns describe feelings of discomfort when discussing finances and even guilt over the cost of care because I often heard the same from experienced veterinarians. After six years in practice, Dr. Dever described her feelings of guilt over finances and euthanasia:

> As medications for animals get better, it gets more expensive to treat animals. Sometimes owners go into debt, and I feel guilty about what it costs. I can't lay the smack down on this guy's owner. My heart really goes out to him because I can tell that this dog is really his buddy. The dog can't move his hind legs, and I was ready to euthanize because I know he doesn't have the money, but the guy says, "Let's see what we can do." I feel horrible because I know that this dog is not going to do the Charleston tomorrow, and I know this will cost the guy more money than he really has. He managed to gather up $500, and I don't want him to spend all this money and the dog not even get better.

Although the veterinarian wanted to help the animal recover from illness, she also believed it important to weigh the cost of treatment against the odds of recovery for the benefit of the owner. Thus, stress comes from the occasional conflict between serving the animal patient and the interests of the client.

Interns were often frustrated when the cost associated with obtaining a diagnosis, such as taking radiographs, getting a blood analysis, or doing exploratory surgery, exceeded what the client was willing or able to pay. Interns feared they would euthanize a sick animal with a treatable problem as Dr. O'Neal explained, "I think the stressful situations are when you can't do the diagnostics so I don't know for sure that this is the right decision. . . . It is something that may be completely treatable, but the owners don't even have the money to find out, so we may be killing treatable animals." Over time, novices like Dr. Jacobs increasingly expressed disappointment and frustration with what some called a fundamental unfairness in financing their patients' care:

> The people who have unlimited resources that they are sinking into this animal—an animal who won't ever walk out of the hospital and won't ever spend another night at home—it is almost kind of the opposite of the other financial problem where they don't have the money to treat. That money could be used to do so much other stuff. You could donate to the shelter or help homeless animals that have broken legs that could easily be fixed, but instead you are just pouring resources into an animal because you can't let it go. To watch one person do that and then to turn around and watch a family put down

a dog because they had to choose between eating and fixing a broken leg—that will always be the worst.

While so many animals in veterinarians' care have to be put down because of a lack of resources, some clients are willing to spend seemingly limitless amounts of money on a few animals with poor prognoses. Novices learn that both types of cases often end in disappointing outcomes for the veterinarian.

Managing the Impression of a Good Death for Clients

As Clinton Sanders notes, client presence during euthanasia can cause difficulties for practitioners, particularly those just beginning their careers.[5] Interns were unanimous that veterinarians must do a good job euthanizing animals because it would be the last memory an owner had of a pet. Interns were fairly confident of their ability to perform the technical aspects of euthanasia, but they reported feeling anxiety that a euthanasia could go wrong in other ways. Some expressed concern that they would cry, and one intern sheepishly recalled a time when he "cried more than the owner" as a student. A resident recalled his early anxieties as an intern: "My main concern was that I didn't want the owners to have a bad experience because of my inexperience in doing it . . . and in saying the right things . . . because it is such an important experience for many of us as pet owners." Although not as looming as their other concerns, lack of experience with client-witnessed euthanasia made the interns quite anxious at the beginning of their internship.

Dealing with Client Emotions

As shown in Chapter 3, veterinarians must deal with the emotions of distressed clients. Novice veterinarians soon recognize that veterinary medicine often involves offering comfort and counsel to clients whose animals they euthanize. Several interns were concerned about time management when it comes to dealing with emotional clients. For example, Dr. Foner had the common worry that his busy caseload would interfere with his ability to attend to the emotional needs of clients: "I think the most challenging will be giving those owners the time and the energy that they need emotionally. I want to always be able to give that, but I've also seen [veterinarians] on emergency . . . [who got] really busy and . . . [attending to clients was] very challenging."

While some interns arrived at their internship after having shadowed residents and been present at euthanasia procedures involving grieving clients, over half had never been present at an owner-witnessed euthanasia. Some clinicians did not allow students in the room during euthanasia as they thought that the student's presence might further upset clients. Even when they were allowed, many interns recalled trying to avoid experiences with emotional clients. Afraid that they would either not know what to say or that they would say the wrong thing, many tried to get out of the room as quickly as possible. If they had no defined role in the process, students often felt as though they were imposing on clients and their grief. Rather than being asked to strictly observe, students preferred to have some role to play such as holding off a vein or restraining an animal. Even minor roles could give them a sense of legitimacy in a situation in which they felt markedly out of place.

When I asked the interns what they took away from watching exchanges during their school years between clinicians and their clients, most reported both positive and negative examples of veterinarian-client interactions. One intern recalled a negative example, a time when she thought a resident was insensitive to a client:

> In school a dog came in that was just wasting away. The owner came in crying because apparently her vet had refused to treat and told her she was being cruel by keeping the dog alive, but my resident also basically told her she was being cruel and that she should euthanize this dog. I don't think that was the right way to deal with that, but I don't know what the right thing to do would have been either.

Most of the interns anticipated feeling awkward or uneasy watching grieving owners and unsure of how to respond to their displays of strong emotion. Dr. Huburt had one such experience during veterinary school: "This woman got really emotional, and it was terrible to watch. So that's hard because it is one of those things that you have to almost be a psychologist or counselor and you have no training for it. I have no idea what to do with these emotionally vulnerable people."

For physicians, especially novice practitioners, communication with patients and relatives when emotions are high is associated with higher levels of stress.[6] Veterinarians and physicians struggle with life-and-death communication, starting from the delivery of bad news[7] to communication regarding the terminally ill.[8] According to surveys of veterinary practitioners, interactions with emotionally distraught owners can be uncomfortable for experienced veterinarians as well as interns.[9] Interns felt especially unprepared to deal with this aspect of their job. As they entered their internships, most felt their formal education failed to adequately prepare them and expressed considerable concern that their skill sets were insufficient to meet the projected emotional demands of the job.

Dealing with Their Own Emotions

Grief over the loss of patients is not unique to veterinary medicine; it is also common to medical professionals caring for humans.[10] Given that many students of veterinary medicine report they went into the profession because they love animals and have had strong bonds with animals throughout their life, it is not surprising that many veterinary professionals experience grief over the loss of patients from time to time.[11] Although interns had varying experiences with grief over the loss of animals in their care as students, they all anticipated they would experience sadness and grief over the loss of patients. Nearly all participants, regardless of experience level, described feeling haunted by the death of some patients and feeling physical signs of grief such as crying, numbness, nausea, tightness in the chest, restlessness, fatigue, insomnia, and appetite disturbance.

Unlike principles of human medicine that assume all patients are in some sense equal in value, there is considerable disagreement about the value of a veterinarian's patients.[12] Not surprisingly, participants often reported that many outsiders did not understand their grief over patients: "So many people can't understand why I get so upset over an animal, especially one that is not even mine, and they don't get why my job can be so hard because they don't value animals like I do." As discussed in Chapter 3, pet owners experience "disenfranchised grief" over the loss of an animal companion, compared to socially recognized grief over loss of a spouse, child, or parent.[13] When veterinarians grieve for the loss of their patients, their grief may also be exacerbated by the social negation of their loss.

Interns at both teaching hospitals where I did my fieldwork expected their internships to be intellectually and physically demanding, but many were also told by professors and friends to expect to do a lot of euthanasia procedures, which induced anxiety in many. Dr. Conrad, like many interns, felt overwhelmed by the frequency of euthanasia during his internship:

> The most challenging aspect of my internship regarding euthanasia, I think, is just the quantity that we have. There were some . . . shifts where I did six or seven in a night. . . . I assumed that there would be a high number of euthanasias, . . . but it is just a lot harder than I thought to actually do them. Something I learned this year is . . . how incredibly prevalent euthanasia is or can be in veterinary medicine.

> You can have, like, five euthanasias in a day—something like that can
> totally get to you. I feel like a murderer because all I have done all day
> is kill things. That doesn't escape you.

Nearly every participant, regardless of how many years in practice, reported feeling stress related to unusually high volume of euthanasias. With over two decades of experience, Dr. Garrett explained that she still feels stress even when she is in agreement that euthanasia is the best course of action: "I will have days go by where nearly every single patient I see I put to sleep. . . . Mostly there's not a whole lot else that we can offer the patient, and . . . the decision to do it is good; I just get tired of doing so many of them—just killing everything I touch."

The prospect of having to kill animals with whom the interns had developed an attachment was a huge concern to them. As they had predicted, by the end of the internship, every intern could recount several times when he or she had an emotional attachment to a euthanized patient. Anticipating that pet owners might choose euthanasia for some patients was agonizing for some interns. At the same time, nearly all the interns expressed concern that they would become jaded to the point that they would no longer be upset over the death of animals and they would lose their ability to empathize with patients and clients. The fear came, in part, from what they perceived as the callous attitude regarding death and euthanasia of the more experienced residents and specialists.

Specific stressors have been associated with the care of terminally ill human patients and their families.[14] For example, physicians wish for a patient's good death—however this is defined—and are disappointed if this does not occur.[15] The same is true for veterinarians. Because attitudes regarding animals vary so widely, veterinarians can find themselves in conflict with clients over the appropriate time and rationale to kill animals. Thus, when the veterinarian is not completely comfortable with the rationale for the patient's death, euthanizing the patient may challenge the veterinarian's identity as a doctor working for the interests of patients—so much so that the veterinarian may feel like an executioner, a murderer, or a killer instead of a doctor. Yet even when a veterinarian is in complete agreement with an owner's decision to euthanize, performing euthanasia can be emotionally difficult.[16]

As interns gained experience, they had trouble adjusting to a role that changed from doing all they could to improve and prolong an animal's life to ending it. Like their physician counterparts,[17] participants often described feeling frustrated at having invested large amounts of energy in caring for patients who then die (sometimes euthanized by the veterinarian). British researchers sent questionnaires to veterinarians asking them how they responded to euthanizing an animal they could not save:[18] 87 percent felt that they were a failure, 67 percent felt depressed, and 46 percent felt guilty. While my study's participants felt guilt and frustration when euthanizing animals they could not save, they often felt worse when the client decided to stop treatment before they were ready to stop. As Dr. Shelly described it: "It is frustrating when owners change their minds or run out of money to treat and . . . all of a sudden they call and say we want to stop . . . and then we have to kill this animal we have been working nonstop to save."

Euthanasia in Veterinary School

Once accepted into veterinary school, students usually complete three years of coursework and then spend most of their final year shadowing clinicians in veterinary hospitals. Within formal clinical environments, students act as aides to experienced veterinarians (interns, residents, and clinicians) caring for hospitalized animals. In addition to the clinical-year experience, many veterinary students worked in veterinary practices before entering school and continue to during summer breaks. Over the past several decades, veterinary schools have been criticized for a lack of formal training related to end-of-life issues; however, a recent survey of the curricula of all twenty-eight veterinary schools in the United States reveals that these trends are changing.[19] Although the level and depth of formal instruction varied widely, most of my study's participants reported at least some coursework related to euthanasia and end-of-life issues, often introduced as a part of a professional ethics, problem-based learning, or client communication course.

Storytelling is an important part of the oral tradition of physician training, although not an official part.[20] The narrative themes tend to focus on sources of stress students face in medical school or those they can anticipate experiencing in a practice. Medical students tell stories about "dog lab"[21] (in which a group of students practice surgeries on an animal over several weeks and then euthanize the animal) and anatomy laboratory[22] but also about undesirable patients, medical error, and accidents.[23] For example, among the many cadaver stories told about anatomy laboratory by physicians in training, one involves incidents in which the cadaver is suddenly revealed to be the mother, uncle, or sixth-grade teacher of the scalpel-wielding student. Frederic Hafferty argues that these stories demonstrate that students can overcome even the most shocking situations.[24]

While sometimes horrific and dark and other times humorous and entertaining, the narratives often have a serious underlying lesson, offering warning to those who disregard the significance of the lesson or fail to take heed.

Erving Goffman calls such cautionary tales "anecdotes from the past" and notes that they serve a variety of purposes: a source of humor, a cathartic expression of anxiety-producing aspects of their job, and disapproval of unacceptable behavior.[25] Nearly every participant in my study could share at least one story heard while in school related to death and dying or euthanasia. Euthanasia-related storytelling falls into two categories, both reflecting the anxieties and concerns of students regarding the real world of veterinary practice: tales of ethically outrageous situations and tales of euthanasia gone wrong.

Ethics-based storytelling reminds students of the ambiguity, contradiction, and paradox in the practice of veterinary medicine. It asks them to anticipate what they would do in a similar situation. Storytellers often present the veterinarians as victims of outrageous adversity and clients' disturbing actions. In the ethically outrageous situations, veterinarians are asked to euthanize animals for what they see as frivolous reasons. In one story a veterinarian was asked to euthanize a client's healthy poodle because poodles are no longer in fashion and she wished to get a more fashionable replacement. The stories of treating animals strictly as property reflect veterinary students' concerns about the ethical dilemmas they will face in the real world.

Some euthanasia-gone-wrong stories involve the unpredictable, strange, or outrageous behavior of clients: "There are folktales out there about clients regretting their decision to euthanize and taking their anger out on the veterinarian by punching him in the face. I don't know if that ever happened, but I think clients can get out of control." Stories of irrational clients are of particular interest to students because they are anxious about dealing with emotional clients and often do not have much experience with them. The general lesson of these stories is to expect the unexpected regarding interactions with clients but that good client communication skills can prevent misunderstandings.

Many of the horror stories focus on animals that do not die after the solution has been administered. In some stories the euthanasia fails because of veterinarian error, but in others the patient can withstand an abnormal amount of solution: "We heard stories where the heart won't stop or you give it an unbelievable amount of medication and the animal still walks around the room." In yet another version of the story, the veterinarian mistakenly believes the animal is dead, but it is only deeply anesthetized: "Everybody has heard the stories where the veterinarian goes into the freezer and hears an animal scratching inside the garbage bag or they give the animal to the owner and it wakes up in the car." Several participants told a similar story, one most had heard in their respective veterinary schools, involving a horse:

INTERN: There are the urban legends of euthanasia like the one where the horse wakes up going down the highway on the flatbed trailer as it is being taken to the rendering plant because the vet did not give enough of the euthanasia solution.

AUTHOR: What do you take away from this story?

INTERN: I don't know if it is true or not, but it seems possible, and I know that I am really going to make sure I give enough solution and the animal is dead. I hear that story but—knock on wood—I have never had one animal come back that I know of [*laughs nervously*].

The stories introduce students to the potential problems and technical challenges of euthanasia.

Other stories that involve technical issues teach students that euthanasia can be unpredictable and the potential for disaster is ever present, especially if certain precautions are not followed. In these stories the owner might be bitten during the euthanasia (usually in the face) or the animal falls off the table while succumbing to the euthanasia solution. Some stories involve medical mistakes such as a careless veterinarian accidentally euthanizing the wrong animal. Researchers find that this sort of storytelling enables doctors to cope with stress and adverse emotions that tend to accompany medical-clinical failure[26] and may even prevent error.[27] Although these tales of disaster might be difficult to hear, the veterinarians involved overcome the disasters and lived to tell the tale. The stories also promote discussion of insider tricks and tactics to help avoid problems and manage technical challenges.

Although mostly legends, these stories present extreme versions of events that do occur in veterinary practice. I should also note that, although these stories were told as true events, I could verify none nor even get two respondents to give the same details. Sometimes the story supposedly happened to someone close to the teller, but names of specific people involved are rarely known. From a sociological perspective, however, I am less concerned with the truth of the stories and more concerned with what they mean for the people who tell them and listen to them. Professional storytelling acts as a teaching tool to help novice practitioners cope with potentially ethically or physically stressful situations. These stories often bonded the group in their mutual horror and sometimes led students to brainstorm creative solutions to potentially challenging future problems.

Although the level and depth of formal and informal instruction varied widely among participants, common themes emerged from the interviews.

Of all of their concerns, interns felt most prepared to handle the technical aspects of euthanasia because those were procedures most interns mastered in clinical contexts. Administering the euthanasia solution involves a routine injection; however, if the intern does not feel confident about hitting a vein, he or she can put in a catheter before the euthanasia to simplify the technical aspect of the procedure. In short, most interns either felt confidence in their ability to handle the technical aspects or saw them as easily manageable with backstage preparation.

In contrast, all interns believed in one way or another that interacting with clients can be complex and unpredictable, requires patience and skill, and involves subtle, conditional aspects rarely made explicit during their schooling. Interns were anxious about giving owners bad news, negotiating the decision to euthanize, discussing financial issues, facing difficult ethical challenges, and dealing with clients' emotions.[28] Although surveys indicate that veterinary students identify these issues related to euthanasia as some of their greatest concerns, veterinary schools have been slow to incorporate training for these into the formal curriculum.[29] Training in work-related skills such as communication, conflict management, and stress management may be helpful when lack of these skills contributes to stress.[30]

As in surveys of other veterinarians, my study's participants complained that their veterinary education placed too much emphasis on the accumulation of information and too little on the ability to think critically and solve real-world problems.[31] Interns' coursework related to ethical decision making and end-of-life issues varied from some to none, but most reported at least some, often introduced as a part of a professional ethics or client communication course. Many participants spoke highly of panels on communication, ethics, and euthanasia in which practitioners were brought in to talk about their experiences in their practice. However, many participants were critical of their ethics-related coursework as lacking realism and social context. Researchers have found evidence for this criticism and argue that the teaching of ethics, for example, could be improved with a focus on the everyday world relevant to practitioners.[32]

Participants often disagreed about the best formats for teaching subjects such as ethical decision making, communication, and end-of-life issues. For example, some practitioners support heavy reliance on clinical instruction, arguing these are skills best learned in the field rather than a classroom: "Everybody can say whatever it is they want to say and how they think they are going to respond in a given situation, but until they get there and they're faced with it, well, it is nothing until you have a family in front of you." Critical of their ethics-related coursework, these veterinarians minimized the practicality of what they learned in the classroom: "We talked about these cases in school, and everybody's got an opinion in the lecture hall of what's right and what's wrong, and that's so stupid. It's so stupid to just sit and talk about it in a room. You don't know how you're going to react when you get there." However, most participants wanted to see more classroom attention given to these topics.

Many scholars of philosophy and biomedical ethics argue in favor of teaching ethical decision making in the classroom because it involves skills that can and should be taught.[33] While research in other medical professions indicates that students can improve their ethical reasoning capabilities through didactic and problem-solving experiences, veterinary students' ethical-reasoning development falls short of these goals.[34] Surveys of the curricula of veterinary medical schools in the United States reveal shortcomings in formal coursework devoted to ethics and ethical decision making.[35] Moreover, Bernard Rollin notes the importance of integrating ethical lessons into the overall curriculum instead of isolating them into one professional ethics course.[36] Yet in some schools, ethical issues associated with end-of-life decision making may be taught only informally during clinical rotations or briefly in conjunction with other subjects such as jurisprudence, professional responsibility, veterinary regulations, and small-animal-practice courses.

Proponents of veterinary communication argue that good communication is essential to a successful veterinary practice and should be taught as part of the formal veterinary curriculum.[37] Research on the teaching of communication in human medicine has demonstrated subsequent improvements in the diagnostic process, medical problem solving, and outcomes of care at all levels of experience.[38] Instruction on end-of-life issues, including relating to patients, can make a positive difference for medical students.[39] Research on veterinary communication suggests that some veterinarians would benefit from improved communication, as they are not fully exploring client concerns or facilitating client involvement in euthanasia decision making.[40]

Unfortunately, few empirical studies examine the effectiveness of various types of communication training in veterinary education. For example, although using trained actors as simulated patients to teach communication skills is well established in human medicine training,[41] it is rarely used in veterinary training and only a few studies have tested the effectiveness for veterinarian-client communication. One study found significant improvement in communication skills of students who received the training compared to control groups.[42] In another study, the use of dramatic scenarios combined with discussion was shown to be more effective than discussion alone.[43] Adding humor to this exercise made it more entertaining than general discussion and the scenarios appeared more realistic to students because they were scripted from actual clinicians' experiences.

For some participants the comfort they offer owners feels natural because they empathize with the humans and the bonds they have with their companion animals, but for others this counseling aspect of the profession is especially challenging. In a study of veterinary students who received pet-loss hotline-support training, students who worked on the hotline reported themselves to be more confident and effective in responding to upset clients compared to those who had no experience on the hotline.[44] Throughout my study, interns, residents, and clinicians continued to experience anxiety and stress related to client counseling and many desired formal training focused on grief management. Surveys of recent veterinary college graduates reveal they are anxious about euthanasia and do not feel competent in delivering bad news or dealing with emotional clients.[45]

While some practitioners call for courses devoted solely to the human-animal bond and grief management to become a standard part of the veterinary curriculum,[46] others argue that this role is outside the domain of knowledge, experience, and responsibility of veterinarians and should not be added to an already full curriculum. Given this disagreement, this book has important implications for veterinary practitioners because it illuminates an often hidden or ignored aspect of the profession. Some veterinarians are actively engaging in the counseling aspects of veterinary medicine (as shown in Chapter 3) with minimal formal training (as shown in this chapter). Although managing client emotions is not generally considered an official aspect of a veterinarian's job, my research suggests that small-animal veterinarians are rethinking old notions of professional responsibility and including managing the emotions of clients whose animals they euthanize.[47] In addition, as shown in Chapter 3, pet owners thanked their veterinarians for providing them comfort and counsel. Studies repeatedly reveal that veterinarians and their clients believe interpersonal skills are one of the most essential characteristics of an effective and successful veterinarian.[48] More specifically, in surveys of client and veterinarian satisfaction regarding the euthanasia experience, both believe that veterinarians should be trained to attend to the emotional needs of the client.[49]

Because dealing with grieving clients is unavoidable, some veterinarians take a more pragmatic view, arguing that grief management might as well be done skillfully and compassionately so that clients will remember this thoughtfulness when it comes time to seek veterinary care for another animal in the future.[50] A sentiment shared among most of my study's participants is that those veterinarians who are more caring and sensitive to the anxieties and emotional needs of clients are better veterinarians and will be more successful in building profitable practices. As demonstrated throughout this chapter, many scholars and veterinary practitioners believe that the skills veterinarians gain from academic coursework help them build profitable practices, improve veterinarian-client relationships, and reduce stress related to ethical decision making, communication, and end-of-life issues.

The Graduates

Veterinary students receive so much more experience with back-stage animal procedures that those procedures become normalized, whereas much of the front-stage work of dealing with clients remains relatively unknown to them (and anxiety producing). In other words, students become familiar with dealing with sick, diseased, and dead animals, whose sights and smells most of the lay public would find disgusting, but they are kept isolated from most interactions and discussions with grief-stricken owners. Thus, looking back over their internship, novices described feeling initially overwhelmed by front-stage matters but gradually becoming more comfortable as they gained experience.

Because the interns valued creating a good last memory for clients (as outlined in Chapter 2), their lack of experience with client-witnessed euthanasia made them anxious. However, as they gained experience, most of the interns became confident in their ability to stage successful euthanasia. Although mistakes happen and technical calamities crop up even for the most seasoned professionals, interns learn techniques to save spoiled performances and create favorable impressions of the death of their patients. By the end of the internship, each intern could list a series of behaviors and skills he or she used to create a good death for animals and a pleasing last memory for the pet owner.

Veterinarians patiently, tirelessly, and daily helped clients deal with the emotional watershed that often accompanies life-and-death decision making. Although dealing with bereaved clients was initially awkward and uncomfortable for most interns, they eventually felt more at ease around emotionally distraught clients. At first, interns were simply reacting to clients' desires and emotions, but they eventually learned to anticipate and deal with clients' emotions (as outlined in Chapter 3). For example, nearly every intern mentioned the need to reassure clients who chose euthanasia for their pets that their choice was appropriate. Although many gradually became more comfortable and competent in this role, others did not.

Time and time again, interns, residents, and more experienced veterinarians told me that one of the first lessons they learned in their internship year was how much of veterinary medicine involved dealing with death and money. Thus, I was not surprised to read that researchers found veterinarians had low confidence specifically in the areas of handling emotional clients and discussing costs of care and payment.[51] Because I repeatedly heard the phrase "Vet school doesn't teach you about death and money," it became crystal clear to me that participants wanted more from their education. Specifically, they wanted to improve their ability to negotiate difficult disagreements with clients, deal with emotional clients, and navigate the business aspects of veterinary medicine. Regardless of their experience level, participants disdained the academic emphasis placed on treating disease while ignoring consideration of the financial realities inherent in the practice of veterinary medicine. They argued that there is no reason that the two cannot be taught in conjunction.

In school, veterinary students are trained to be medical providers to animal patients, but in the real world they have to learn a customer orientation. Young students idealistically believed that finances should be separated from treatment decisions, but over time they understood that cost influences the type of treatment chosen.[52] As they gained clinical experience, interns became better at talking with clients about financing patient care; however, negotiating the cost of treatment still felt frustrating, difficult, and distasteful at times. Most come to accept it as part of the job. For example, weighing an uncertain outcome against the cost of treatment no longer provokes the distress it did for some interns in the beginning: "People love numbers. They always want to know what the chances are . . . you know, what are the odds? It bothered me at first to boil a patient's life down to some number, but it is important to for clients who have to make tough choices."

Few of the interns had developed strong enough personal values to completely withstand the psychological stress of their internship, and many had their idealism shattered, as the reality of the job was not what they imagined:

You are this empathetic animal-adoring person, and suddenly your job is to euthanize this animal you have never met before, for this person you have never met before who is falling apart with emotion. But they are also asking you to do something against your beliefs. They are not these evil people, and their stories are more complicated than you imagined when you were in school. You have this vision of what it is going to be like as a veterinarian, and you think you have solid standards of what you will do and what you won't do, and you are going to be as good as anybody and maybe even better than all of them. But the reality is that you have to deal with what comes to you, and it is never all that straightforward. This is something that you have to learn how to deal with, and you eventually ease your way into this act of the profession.

Several acted in ways they would later regret such as euthanasia of an animal at the owner's request that they believed was not justified. Others regretted that they had "allowed owners to keep animals alive too long," resulting in the unnecessary suffering of their patients. Interns would frequently cry when asked to recall these situations, holding on to strong feelings even after several months' time. The frustration of interns was often compounded by astonishment and dismay as they realized how far from their initial ideals they or their fellow interns would venture.

Veterinary interns experience personal responsibility and workload that is unprecedented in their experience. Working extraordinarily long hours, some interns had difficulty maintaining their initial ideals: "I hate to admit it but in some cases where I sort of want to argue with them . . . I just go ahead and do what they want because it can be easier and I haven't slept in days and [then] I get to go home." In a similar circumstance, this intern felt as though suppressing her moral principles was sometimes an inevitable part of her demanding schedule and busy caseload:

> It feels terrible when you don't have time to convince an owner not to euthanize and you try to explain to them that it is a treatable disease. Things crash, and there are four emergencies waiting for you, and you don't have time to deal with them and really talk to them about it. When they make that decision and I could have changed their mind and I don't have time to talk to them so I am like "Okay let's go," I just [euthanize] the animal and get back to my other cases. [*Eyes tearing.*] That weighs on me. I just don't think many of us can avoid it and get what we need to do done.

Interns sometimes justified their behavior as practical so they could have time to concentrate on the other animals in their care.

Exhausted from working long hours, a couple of interns felt as though they acted against their moral principles by pushing clients toward euthanasia to avoid difficult cases:

> I've felt like, you know, there was a period during the internship where I was like, "It's just easier for me to [*sighs*]—to get these people to put their dog to sleep than it is for me to—to deal with it all, over and over again." But I think that that's probably what you'll see

is that that happens. I mean, they were mostly dying anyway, and you just wanted to have something that was easy and straightforward and something you—you didn't have to book in [for treatment], so sometimes you just present it in such a way that you know they will choose euthanasia.

You look at the dying cat with cancer on the list and you are like, "Ugh, if they wanted to book this in, it would be days, and we would be running so many tests, and it would be so much work" on top of the eight hundred other problems you are trying to solve as an intern. So when those people who bring that dog in that can't walk, that has heart failure and renal failure and now has an ulcer and has all these problems, I may word it in such a way that they euthanize right away. That is not something pleasant to think about, but it is true. I have never [exactly] lied . . . , but I have presented it in such a way that I am trying to push them towards that.

Although interns might have felt as though they were pushing clients, to my knowledge they never withheld information or intentionally deceived them into choosing euthanasia. Yet virtually all the participants reported stress when thinking back on certain cases—wondering whether they encouraged own-ers to choose euthanasia for the wrong reasons. Feelings of guilt were more intense if the veterinarian had at some point become frustrated with diffi-cult illnesses or clients. Interns clearly struggled to adjust to the legitimate demands of balancing their exhausting schedules with quality patient care.

Organizational pressures led participants to compromise their ethical standards. Interns, constantly under pressure to prove themselves to supervi-sors, for example, reported difficulty following their moral principles that went against the stated or assumed wishes of their superiors. They sometimes went along with morally questionable behavior without protest for fear of damaging relationships that could negatively influence their careers.[53] This intern, under nearly around-the-clock pressure from supervisors, described using euthanasia as an easy solution to potentially problematic interactions with supervisors:

If you have a lot of euthanasias, that will get you down. But if you have really been hounded by a resident or something, that can be bad too. . . . Sometimes when you are new and just starting out with difficult cases, you may feel that euthanasia is a way out of problems because it is easier than figuring things out sometimes—when you are constantly in the grind of an internship, and everyone is always questioning you on everything, and you always feel like you are either in over your head or kind of swamped or drowning or being criticized.

By blaming their demanding schedules and difficult supervisors, interns justified violating their ethical principles.

For most novice interns, their ethical principles remained the same, but the details were rewritten. For example, most interns held firm in their disapproval of euthanasia for the convenience of clients, but their definition of what constituted convenience changed over time. Just a month into his internship, Dr. Jacobs defined his feelings on convenience euthanasia:

> Anytime an animal might need an inhaler for asthma or some kind of bronchitis, some people just freak out about it. To me that is a reason of convenience. Actually another good one would be giving the sub-Q [subcutaneous] fluids at home or insulin. There are some people that just are not comfortable with it. They always say, "Isn't there just a pill? Do I really have to give an injection every single day? Do I really have to give it every time, the same time every day? How annoying!" Well, I say *they* are annoying. I just won't do those where it is just the convenience of the owner.

Like many interns, Dr. Jacobs narrowed his definition of convenience euthanasia as his internship progressed, which meant he did more euthanasias. What is most interesting about Dr. Jacobs is that by the end of his internship he excluded every example he had initially listed from his definition of *convenience euthanasia*. For instance, he no longer considered it a reasonable expectation that the client give the pet a daily injection. Calling his old definition "naive," Dr. Jacobs's new limits were considerably narrowed: "I won't do those 'I'm moving' convenience ones or the allergies-in-the-family thing." Concepts that seemed so clear and transparent to novices at the beginning of the year became dense and complicated as the year progressed.

Many interns came to see their initial definitions as naive and their new ones as realistic and practical. Like Dr. Jacobs, many of the interns who initially thought they would never euthanize a diabetic patient began to see cases where pet owners were not conscientious and the patient suffered. Dr. Green described how her definition of diabetes as a treatable and reasonably manageable disease changed as a result of her clinical experience:

> It is not a wrong decision to euthanize that animal, because without that treatment—for whatever reason, like, the cat is too bad or clients don't have time—the animal can get much more sick and suffer a

lot more. You only have to see so many animals in diabetic shock to change your mind on this issue. It is not worth it to me if the owners are not 100 percent committed—I don't push it anymore. This is where, depending on the owner, a treatable disease is no longer treatable.

At the end of her internship, Dr. Green said, "I always have to remind myself that it is better to be euthanized than to die an uncomfortable death from a treatable disease." In the beginning many novices were surprised that some owners were unwilling to make for pets what interns considered minimal effort. However, they began to see a wide range of pet owners, some whose willingness to do necessary care at home exceeded their expectations and others who disappointed.

When it comes to managing ethical uncertainty, much of the literature supports a concept of cognitive dissonance, a term used to describe the disparity between people's attitudes and their actions.[54] The theory is that people strive for internal consistency between beliefs and behavior, and the greater the distance between the two, the greater the effort they have to make to avoid strain. People respond to cognitive dissonance by either changing their attitudes or by modifying their behavior. By having malleable attitudes, interns were able to remain true to their initial ethical principles. Redefining concepts such as convenience for many young veterinarians neutralized the cognitive dissonance they initially had and helped them avoid seeing their actions as immoral.

Researchers studying idealism traced the fate of the meaning of *public interest law* among law students and found that graduating seniors believed they emerged from school with their altruism intact.[55] However, researchers documented that the students' concept of public interest law changed over the years and held very different meanings for incoming and graduating students. Like young lawyers, many interns revised their definitions of *health* and *illness* as their first year progressed:

I never put down a healthy animal, but my definition of *healthy* has changed. Maybe that is how I keep my ethics in check so that I can say I have never euthanized a healthy animal. My ethics didn't change . . . , but I became more *realistic* in my definition of healthy. If the animal doesn't get the necessary treatment, they will suffer and they will die from a so-called treatable disease. If the client doesn't have the funds, a treatable disease becomes a terminal disease.

Like both the previous interns, many said that they would never euthanize a healthy animal, but their definitions of *healthy* and *terminal illness* changed in such a way that they were able to keep their original moral principles with fewer ethical conflicts. Novices were able to hold on to their initial ideals by redrawing boundaries around certain concepts.

The scientific ideology inherent in veterinary training often denies that science makes any value judgments, but the meanings of *health, disease,* and *sickness* are heavily influenced by values. Many concepts related to health and illness, such as quality of life, are not empirically obvious properties and their definitions vary considerably from veterinarian to veterinarian. When asked to list the criteria they use to evaluate quality of life for their patients, veterinarians gave widely different accounts:

> I find that a lot of veterinarians base it on whether or not the pet is eating. Me, personally, I don't think that that is really the only thing that you need to look at, 'cause I have seen several pets that owners don't want to put to sleep because they have a great appetite but the dog still can't walk and is blind and deaf and has a number of medical problems. But just because he is still eating, I don't necessarily still consider their quality of life to be good.

Some veterinarians focus solely on the physical attributes of animals; others include psychological traits as well. Yet even when two veterinarians agree as to the exact set of characteristics that count as good measure of quality of life, they may then disagree as to how to evaluate and measure those characteristics. For example, many veterinarians believed euthanasia was always acceptable for suffering animals, but definitions of *pain* or *discomfort* varied considerably from veterinarian to veterinarian.

The original ethical beliefs and values that the interns brought with them to the internship were far from immutable, and interns were able to hold on to their initial ideals and reconcile internal moral conflict by redefining ethical principles. For example, the practice of euthanasia influenced some interns to rethink other ethically challenging practices such as onychectomy,[56] or cat declawing: "The option of euthanasia changes things. Because of euthanasia I think differently today about practices in veterinary medicine than I did before I started working . . . take declawing, for example. Declawing can be a life-saving procedure! I used to think I would *never* declaw a cat. Now if the owner is going to put the animal down because it scratches the furniture, I will declaw the cat rather than euthanize it." This veterinarian resolved an initially ethically challenging situation by redefining it as a life-saving procedure.

Over the last few decades, many veterinary journals have featured articles on ethical issues in the provision of veterinary services, and those associated with end-of-life issues and euthanasia are prominent.[57] As they were leaving their internship, many interns continued to struggle with reconciling conflicts that sometimes occur between personal values and patient or professional demands. Veterinarians are burdened with the task of deciding not only what counts as a legitimate rationale to dispense death but also how to define the evidence to establish this claim. And different veterinarians will often take entirely different approaches to the same issue. One veterinarian may perceive the killing of an animal with diabetes as unacceptable killing of a healthy animal, but another may see it as a terminal disease in which euthanasia is a legitimate option because of the burden on the pet owner.

M ost of the interns identified euthanasia as presenting some of the most challenging aspects of their internship. This is not surprising, as end-of-life decision making often involves high emotions, clinical unpredictability, and choices between equally unfavorable options. Interns often faced dilemmas that pitted their idealism against pragmatism, in which what they wanted to do conflicted with what was more practical, what an owner could afford, or what others wanted or expected of them. Doing what appeared right to them at times seemed to conflict with doing what was most practical for their patient:

> I think it is difficult for interns to learn the pragmatic way of practicing medicine. Right out of vet school you are taught the best medicine, and you get to do the best medicine. At first I would approach these cases . . . I would always present the ideal way to fix things, and I think I did get slapped in the face a few times and shocked by owners who have nothing and they can't proceed at all so we euthanized. I learned to feel out each situation, and I have started to give more options. Give the best option first and I say that "this is ideal and what is best for your pet," and then I say, "Or you could give something a bit more middle of the line a try. It is not ideal, but it is affordable and practical." You have to let go of always doing everything and doing the best if you want to avoid euthanizing everything that walks in the door.

Many interns began to feel that defining patients' health and quality of life was not always as clear-cut as they would prefer. The decision to euthanize an animal is a complex, negotiated process between client and veterinarian.

This phenomenon of reality shock, which often happens as novices confront the inconsistencies between their dreams of the profession and what it is really like, has been reported in many occupations, especially medicine and law.[58] Although some novices suffer stress and loss of self-esteem, most adopt the coping strategies common to their profession (as discussed in Chapter 5) to deal with the distress they feel. From human-medicine students[59] to police officers training to become members of the animal-cruelty investigation unit,[60] as novices encounter the dilemmas of the real world, their idealism takes a serious hit. However, over time, another kind of optimism develops—one tempered by the reality of the job, which allows workers to face the necessary challenges and to derive satisfaction, reward, and happiness from their work.

Veterinary novices come to realize that moral issues are embedded in messy, real-life situations that involve weighing the animal's interests against those of the client. While some veterinarians are clearly more client oriented and others more patient centered, most seem to strive for balance. At the end of the year, I asked participants who were seasoned interns what advice they would give the new incoming-intern cohort. They almost exclusively focused on the importance of considering multiple perspectives and being morally flexible in their work—both with clients and colleagues. On one hand, they would encourage new recruits to keep an open mind to the owner's point of view, try to see things from their perspective, and try not to judge their decisions. On the other hand, interns also wanted to inspire the newbies to advocate for their patients, to educate the owners on behalf of animals, and to resist pressure to do things that make them uncomfortable. Using the metaphor of a bridge designed to withstand powerful wind, one intern said, "Be flexible, but don't break."

5

Coping with Euthanasia

Emotion-Management Strategies

All veterinary encounters are carefully negotiated, triangular interactions involving the veterinarian, the human client, and the animal patient. Because the animal is nonverbal and basically powerless to participate in any consultation, the client and veterinarian must determine the animal's problem and negotiate an outcome for the patient.[1] As both service providers to their human clients and medical professionals to their animal patients, the divided responsibilities can be difficult for veterinarians to balance, causing them difficult ethical dilemmas.[2] As seen in Chapter 1, conflicts between veterinarians and their clients can occur for many reasons. For example, veterinarians may differ from their clients in personal values and opinions regarding the ethical treatment of animals.

This chapter is concerned with emotional and moral stress associated with animal death and the practice of euthanasia. Veterinary work causes distress for practitioners because it requires people who care strongly for animals to kill them, often when they are not sick enough to easily justify their death. The philosopher Bernard Rollin argues that animal-care professionals are exposed to a unique type of euthanasia-related moral stress.[3] As described by Rollin, animal-care professionals typically enter their occupations because they want to help animals but then face a contradiction between what they believe they ought to be doing (e.g., protecting animals) and the reality of what they are asked to do (e.g., kill animals).[4] Consistent with Rollin's notion of moral stress, Arnold Arluke uses the term *caring-killing paradox* to describe how animal-care professionals experience emotional stress when they are expected to euthanize animals for whom they have provided care and protection.[5]

In addition to this kind of euthanasia-related stress, veterinarians bear another conflicting responsibility related to end-of-life care, the duty to protect patients from unnecessary suffering and the obligation to continue life support as requested by pet owners. The veterinarian's technical expertise and the client's intimate attachment to the animal can lead them to different conclusions regarding the best interest of the animal. How do they do these tasks without abandoning a sense of themselves as people who work in the best interest of animals? How do veterinarians resolve challenging situations, manage ethical uncertainty, and deal with uncomfortable feelings?

The stress literature identifies two basic types of coping strategies: problem focused and emotion focused.[6] Problem-focused tactics involve mobilizing actions aimed to change the realities of the situation. The techniques veterinarians rely on to resolve disagreements with clients outlined in Chapter 1 are primarily problem-focused approaches. Emotion-focused tactics typically involve regulating one's emotions linked to the stressful situation without necessarily changing the reality of that situation. Thus, the emotion-focused coping strategies outlined in this chapter are more concerned with adapting to stressors rather than changing them. While problem-focused coping would seem most effective because it directly addresses the cause of the distress, Susan Folkman and Richard Lazarus suggest both strategies may be necessary because overcoming problematic emotions is often related to overcoming the problem.[7]

The effectiveness of problem-focused coping, of course, depends on whether the stressor is controllable.[8] Stressors associated with veterinary euthanasia involve both controllable and uncontrollable events. Whatever the level of stress my study's participants experienced, which depended to some extent on personal values, all relied on both problem- and emotion-focused coping tactics. As outlined in Chapter 1, veterinarians use problem-focused strategies to negotiate disagreements with clients. However, these tactics do not always resolve the problem. In this chapter I first briefly outline the imperfections in problem-focused strategies before moving on to the emotion-focused strategies veterinarians use to manage their emotions and resolve ethical uncertainty. The chapter concludes by investigating problems implementing emotion-focused strategies, exploring why some people do not consistently use them and why they sometimes fail to resolve tensions.

Imperfections in Problem-Focused Strategies

Problem-focused strategies often helped veterinarians avoid stress related to euthanasia but did not always change the outcome for the animal, thus falling short for veterinarians. For example, the strategy of convincing pet owners to surrender their animals to local animal shelters could avoid euthanasia. However, Dr. Spencer, as did many participants, feared that less-than-perfect animals would unhappily spend the remainder of their lives in crowed shelters and end up euthanized anyway:

> In the beginning I would have been more likely to try to get them to surrender. Like if they would come in and say, "Oh, he is old, and he pees on the rug, but maybe the shelter can adopt out a dog like that?" No, . . . no one will want to adopt it, so it will get euthanized, and it will spend its last two weeks uncomfortable in a shelter environment.

Sometimes participants did not want to ask the shelter to take on more animals—especially those perceived as unadoptable—because they felt sorry for shelter workers who have to euthanize so many animals. As a problem-focused strategy, surrendering animals to a local shelter can provide a good alternative for relatively healthy, young, and well-behaved animals because they have the best chance of adoption. However, a nagging skepticism sometimes diminished the positive feeling of hope that the strategy would give the animal a chance for adoption.

The veterinarian in some instances faces legal obligations to follow the wishes of the owner. One of the most difficult disagreements between veterinarians and their clients involved owners who wished to continue treating or artificially sustaining the life of their terminally ill companion animal despite the animal's poor prognosis. According to an American Veterinary Medical Association legal brief, veterinarians' right to terminate service is far more limited than their clients' right to take their animal and leave:

> Clients, our courts have said, do not have to accept professional service from anyone any longer than they desire. The health professional, on the other hand, must continue service once the contract is created until the result has been achieved or until he can voluntarily terminate it without injury to the client. As a matter of law, it is generally stated that if a professional wishes to discontinue service, he should not do so during any critical phase in the rendition of such service.[9]

The problem for veterinarians is that they could not refer these clients to other veterinarians because the patients are gravely ill and transfer is likely to cause death. In these cases, veterinarians feel a strong duty to protect patients from unnecessary suffering and they may even wryly joke about accidentally slipping the patient the blue juice. However, intentionally inducing the death of animal against the owner's wishes is highly unethical, and participants were duty bound to continue life support as requested by pet owners despite how upsetting it could be for them. Many participants described these types of disagreements with clients as some of the worst to resolve.

Although a veterinarian has the legal right to refuse requests for euthanasia, many felt guilty doing so because their refusal only shifted responsibility to a fellow colleague or local animal shelter. Many veterinary practices have policies regulating veterinarian refusal of clients' requests. At some hospitals, administrators strongly discourage veterinarians from refusing owners' requests, believing that it is a veterinarian's responsibility to carry out owners' wishes. Other hospitals encouraged veterinarians to act as their conscience dictated. A veterinarian's stress can be exacerbated when employed in a practice with colleagues whose moral views do not match his or her own: "I have had a huge problem when it comes to the front desk and euthanasia; . . . they get mad when we don't want to euthanize. . . . You don't need someone to make you feel bad about it or make you defend your decision."

Killing sick animals with good prognoses simply for financial reasons was often the most difficult euthanasia procedure to avoid. Rarely, animal shelters or rescue organizations have special funds to cover medical expenses, but these funds are generally quite limited. Dr. Sanchez explained the difficulties of problem-focused strategies in these cases:

> Say the dog is sick, but certainly fixable, and it would cost three or four thousand, and the moral dilemma for me is you can't require people to just cough up three or four thousand. That is not a fair expectation, and that is not the way we should practice medicine. Yes, ideally, but you can't just say you are an asshole for not wanting to pay three or four thousand for your pet. It is a lot of money, so if they are really sick and the treatment is going to be expensive, then unfortunately, euthanasia does become an option. . . . It is also not the kind of thing where we can surrender him [to an animal shelter without treating him first].

Some veterinary hospitals and clinics set aside small funds so that employees can do medical treatments pro bono; however, alternatives to euthanasia often require more substantial funds. If the treatment exceeds the set limit, the policy may allow the veterinarian to treat the animal free of charge but generally requires pet owners to surrender ownership, and the animal is placed in a new home. Offering services for free or reduced prices is not a viable problem-based strategy because veterinarians cannot make a habit of this if they expect to stay in business.

Even when problem-based strategies avoided the original cause of the stressor, veterinarians often felt tremendous stress related to the strategy itself. Dr. Miller described how pro bono work avoids the stress of financially based euthanasia but can be heartrending for the veterinarian who has to watch distraught pet owners reluctantly sign over custody: "It is so hard to take the pet from them when they are sobbing. . . . It sucks to take this kid's dog away, to take anyone's pet away, when they can't afford treatment, but I sure wasn't going to kill the dog." Some clients regret their decision and have accused the veterinarian of stealing their animal. If their pro bono work required surrender, some participants did not invoke this strategy because taking the animal away from the pet owners was so emotionally upsetting. When participants did use the strategy, they felt good to have saved their patient but felt cruel to their clients: "I feel like a total asshole, but . . . there are two options: either it is your pet and you pay the deposit, or it is not your pet anymore."

Problem-focused coping worked best to resolve some straightforward disagreements with clients but offered little help with ethical dilemmas, difficult situations with no clearly preferable outcome. When it comes to life-and-death decisions veterinarians must deal with an array of ethical dilemmas. Decisions regarding euthanasia of companion animals are rarely straightforward because they often require consideration of factors beyond the health and comfort of the animal. For example, when a hundred-pound, arthritic bullmastiff experiences increasing difficulty walking up and down stairs to the client's third-floor apartment, euthanasia may be decided on because of the demands on the owner.

Sometimes the veterinarian's problem-focused strategies to resolve disagreements with the client were unsuccessful. In some cases, veterinarians agreed to their client's request because they were unable to negotiate a better alternative for the animal or pet owner. Others ended in favorable outcomes for patients but came with a hefty moral or emotional cost to the veterinarian. As we saw in Chapter 1, lying to clients may sway them to the veterinarian's desire, but such a strategy violates the veterinarian's professional ethical code. Participants sometimes broke their hospital's pro bono policies, but this strategy risks reprimand and damaging relationships with colleagues. Even if problem-focused strategies ended favorably, the negotiation process itself was often emotionally draining.

Emotion-Management Strategies

Emotional Distancing: Animals as Pets and Patients

Getting emotionally attached to patients adds to any veterinarian's difficulties when he or she is called on to end the patient's life. Like many other participants, Dr. Petrich managed uncomfortable feelings over euthanasia by making a distinction between a *patient* and an anonymous *pet*:

> [Performing euthanasia] is certainly different for patients that we have worked with a lot, but when you don't really know them, it is just another thing that is on the list that has to be done. . . . It is not really as—I don't want to say "emotional" because it is, but it is different for a *patient* or *just someone's pet* that is old and sick and [that it's] time to euthanize. (Emphasis added)

As Dr. Petrich's statement demonstrates, veterinarians felt more emotionally prepared for the death of animals brought in specifically for euthanasia. As veterinary students, some interns had distanced themselves from grief over the loss of an animal by not thinking of them as their patients: "Animals in clinics haven't really been my patients. And I haven't worked hard and tried to make them feel better or been the one to manage their care. So I really haven't had that attachment." Thus, as in Dr. Edwards's experience, veterinarians create boundaries to establish emotional distance from animals: "In your mind you are putting together one plan versus the other. [Either] [t]he animal . . . becomes your patient and you treat him, or you euthanize him. You just click it into place when they make their decision."

Like shelter workers, veterinarians protect themselves against emotional involvement by avoiding attachments to animals for whom euthanasia seemed likely.[10] For example, as Dr. O'Neal explained, if the animal's medical care required expensive treatment, participants tried to evaluate whether clients would be willing or able to invest the necessary funds or would choose euthanasia:

> If it is over a certain amount of money, I often assume they are not going to treat or be able to pay for treatment. . . . If [the animals] are not vaccinated or they are full of fleas or ticks or have untreated wounds, I guess there are certain red flags that you pick up on that you make an assumption this person is not going to invest anything. You can feel that they don't seem to put effort into their animal. . . . Sometimes they surprise you and make the investment. Not very often, but they

do. It just helps when you know not to get your hopes up so you can just not get that attached to the animal.

Similarly, residents commonly asked their interns to estimate the likelihood of treatment: "This is a $1,200 cat. Do you think the owners will go for it?" If the intern believed treatment is likely, residents spent time assessing the case and sketching out a plan for the "patient." However, if the intern was doubtful the clients would pursue life-saving treatment, the resident gave comparatively little notice to the "pet" and moved to the next case. By anticipating from the beginning whether the pet owner is unable or unwilling to pay for alternatives to euthanasia, the veterinarian can avoid getting too attached to the animal.

Virtually all of the novice interns feared that they would be hurt or burn out if they could not achieve some level of emotional detachment. Emotional detachment was not always easy to achieve for many novices, and for some interns it was a considerably difficult task. Yet for others, emotional distance seemed to come with relative ease. In Spencer Cahill's study of mortuary science students, he noticed that many seemed better able to achieve the necessary emotional distance compared to some of their peers (and him).[11] The students who were able to more quickly adjust to emotionally challenging aspects of dealing with the dead all had family members in the funeral business, leading Cahill to argue that those students entered school with emotional capital that others lacked. Similarly, the attitudes and values of veterinarians regarding animals are influenced by their experiences in childhood and adolescence.

In line with Cahill, a few of my study's participants suggested that it was easier for them to keep emotional distance because of their background—such as growing up on a farm, in a geographically rural area, or in another culture. Dr. Stevens described his early life and experiences with animals in Lebanon, before he moved to New York in his adolescence. He said, "When I have to euthanize something that really shouldn't be euthanized, it is not as hard for me as it is for some of my colleagues." When I asked him why, he credited his family background:

I never had pets growing up. My dad is from Jordan, and my mom is from Lebanon . . . so just the idea of having an animal in the house is kind of odd to them. Animals were not really companions but were for some use. The cats that they might have considered pets are like stray cats that you feed and that is it. . . . People are less willing to spend as much money on animals. . . . I guess it makes it easier to recommend euthanasia . . . [when clients] can't afford something or whatever reason because of spending time in Lebanon and thinking about how animals are treated differently there.

Dr. Kaufman, who grew up in Israel, described a similar outlook on pet animals: "If you have a dog, it is outside, and that's just where animals belong, is outside, so we don't have *pets*—I mean, they don't belong on a bed or in a living room." Although today her dogs share her bed, she believed her early experiences made it easier for her—compared to peers with different backgrounds—to create emotional distance from patients.

Common themes emerged among participants who felt they brought something akin to Cahill's emotional capital with them to the job. Unlike nearly all of their peers, many had not developed emotional connections to animals until their adulthood. They hypothesized that they were more accustomed to being around people who had a strictly utilitarian approach to nonhuman animals compared to their peers: "Where I grew up it's all mostly what the animal will do for you; . . . cows, goats, horses . . . do things for you and they work for you." With regard to companion animals, Dr. Cartwright provided a statement representative of those who grew up on a farm or in a rural area: "It is simply different in the Midwest. . . . People get attached to pets there, but if Fluffy gets sick, they are more likely to think, 'We can just get a new dog and spend this money on something else.' They aren't cold people or heartless at all, but they just see things differently." Although they too struggled at times to achieve emotional distance, these practitioners believed their background helped them see animals in their care as both subjects and objects, "patients" and "property."

Some novices feared that emotional distancing might cause them to become jaded or burned out and they would not be the kind of caring, sympathetic veterinarian they wanted to become. Abortion clinic counselors similarly struggle to create the necessary emotional distance to get the job done but fear going too far, such that they would no longer be able to authentically help people: "If they stayed invested in their work, then they experienced a host of negative emotions that made work tiring and stressful. If they detached, then they felt they were not effectively providing care."[12] Veterinary students, as in many other occupations that rely on emotional distancing as a coping strategy, are expected to learn a careful balancing act.

Veterinarians with decades of experience often nostalgically recalled the more intense attachments they felt for the animals in their care as younger practitioners. However, they also recalled that those unguarded emotional attachments come with a hefty cost. For example, Dr. Baker, a veterinarian with over thirty years' experience, told me that he used to let himself get "all wrapped up" in a case. These early experiences were an "emotional roller-coaster ride," in which he would get incredibly excited at a patient's slightest improvement and extremely depressed when conditions worsened. Although he valued the connections he continues to develop with patients, he is undeniably more guarded: "Now I don't let myself get too wrapped up. . . . I find myself more distant. . . . I think this is what happens to veterinarians as they gain more and more experience."

Like their human-medicine counterparts,[13] veterinary students are taught that complete detachment can lead to a lack of concern for patients but that getting too close to patients can compromise their medical judgment and the quality of care. But today's human patients and veterinary clients want to feel as though they are in the hands of professionals who care about their or their pet's well-being. Emotion and connection should thus be sparse and balanced with detachment. Talcott Parsons describes this seemingly incongruous mind-set as "affective neutrality,"[14] while Renee Fox prefers the term "detached concern."[15] The blending of counterattitudes, "detachment" with "concern," is nothing new to medical training, as students are taught to balance idealism with realism, uncertainty with certainty, and self-orientation with other-orientation.[16]

During their internships, novice veterinarians are expected to learn to balance detachment with concern. On one hand, supervisors considered it important that interns not become desensitized to the feelings and emotions of their patients or indifferent to the killing of animals. Interns are told to "remember what you are here for" and "why you got into this profession in the first place." On the other hand, supervisors warned interns that extreme attachment could cloud their judgment, leading them to make bad medical decisions. Interns are advised to build a protective emotional callus and put up walls around their emotions: "When you just don't have that little callus, . . . then it hits you a little harder."

By the time novices enter their internship, they do not have to be told they are expected to develop emotional detachment; they were warned, during clinical rotations in school, not to get too attached. Moreover, some lab exercises create distance from animals. Like human-medicine education,[17] veterinary education often includes using living dogs to illustrate basic physiology principles, after which the dogs are killed.[18] Although this practice has become quite controversial[19] (and is discussed in the Conclusion in greater detail), many veterinary and medical schools defend the use of "dog lab." Sociologically speaking, the laboratory exercise has the effect of distancing veterinary students from their patients, who learn to see dogs in the laboratory as learning tools rather than patients.

Emotional distance is also achieved, in part, by learning to think of the animal as a series of technical puzzles to be solved rather than as a patient with feelings. Interns often introduced their patients to me according to the type of specialty surgery they expected to learn, such as "my hip replacement" or "my soft tissue sarcoma surgery." When among fellow insiders, participants of all experience levels frequently referred to patients by their disease or medical problem rather than their name. For example, patients were introduced as "my hemangiosarcoma" or "my prolapsed eye." A dog with severe, advanced abdominal cancer was even comically introduced as "a stomach tumor with a dog attached."

Despite emotionally distancing techniques that encouraged veterinarians to see animals as objects, animals were also seen as individuals worthy of compassion and sympathy with feelings and desires. The culture of the teaching hospital is that it is normal and expected for veterinarians to be touched by the suffering and death of animals as well as by the grief of their clients. As seen in earlier chapters, veterinarians show genuine (and sometimes intense) sympathy and are sensitive to their patient's comfort and the owner's grief. Participants filled their desks and workspaces with photos of favorite patients or patients they had euthanized along with letters and cards from owners thanking them for their support. While showing me collections of patient photos, some participants openly cried and others choked backed tears as their voices cracked.

The hope, of course, is that veterinary professionals learn to accommodate these emotions so that they do not become overly strained or emotionally burned out. Yet at times participants became so attached to their patients that they were overwhelmed with emotion when anticipating their death. Even with patients they had just met, veterinarians often felt great sadness at the prospect of euthanizing them. Nearly all participants believed it was important to have some emotional distance, but they also valued their connections to patients and clients. By learning to balance detachment with concern, veterinarians were able to maintain an emotionally safe distance yet not entirely detach themselves from the patient.[20]

Emotional Distancing: Humor, Slang, and Laughter

As mentioned in the Introduction, participants sometimes employed dark humor to create emotional distance from death and cope with death-related situations. Veterinarians used humor, slang, and laughter in multiple contexts for a variety of purposes. During my research, I was struck by the volume of humorous exchanges in day-to-day banter as well as the number of pranks and practical jokes. For example, veterinarians enjoyed playing pranks on clients by putting pink casts on the broken legs of tough-looking, male pit bulls, rottweilers, and bulldogs. Participants clearly relished the incongruous image of their patients as well as the owner's expression: "You should have seen the look on that guy's face! I love doing that. It always gets a laugh."

Veterinarians regularly poke fun at the silly or cute antics of animals, but they more often joke about disgusting puss-filled wounds and flea-ridden, flatulent patients. Like nurses,[21] medical students,[22] emergency responders,[23] and prison officers,[24] veterinarians and their technicians[25] use humor when dealing with the physically dirty tasks of their profession, including dealing with dead bodies, unpleasant odors, blood, excrement, and vomit. Through self-deprecating humor, all of these workers were able to characterize themselves as a special group of people capable of withstanding the physically and emotionally dirty aspects of the occupation. Because such work can seem ridiculous, demeaning, and stigmatizing, humor provides distance from the offending task and helps turn a disgusting situation into something more bearable.

Laughter and joking among insiders often creates a sense of unity, ameliorates the strain of common problems, builds rapport among staff, and strengthens their morale.[26] From physicians[27] to prostitutes,[28] workers engage in derogatory jokes that mock problematic patients and clients. Veterinarians are no exception. In Clinton Sanders's study of problematic veterinary clients, some clients were the subject of jokes because they were seen by veterinarians as "so hopelessly ignorant of the basic requirements of animal caretaking that they were viewed with sort of sad bemusement."[29] A favorite backroom pastime of my study's participants involved regaling colleagues with amusing stories about crazy, peculiar, anxious, or high-maintenance clients. Indeed, some especially entertaining tales reached near folklore status around the hospital. As far as I could confirm, one story, involving an eccentric client who strolled her elderly beagle around the hospital in a baby carriage, could be traced back nearly twenty years.

Clients seen as irresponsible or neglectful pet owners were often the subject of joking and ridicule. For example, Dr. Brown's scorn for some clients was clear in her sarcastic remarks, such as "We see a lot of [clients whose pets fell from] high-rise [windows] . . . in New York. These people are annoying. You can spend $2 on a screen or $2,000 at the [hospital]. What sounds better to you? What morons!" Clients deemed ignorant of their animal's serious condition were also the subject of contempt. For example, upon telling his colleagues that his patient had been "breathing funny for a week," the veterinarian sarcastically added, "Wow, they rushed her right in!" Another participant mocked client negligence by portraying the "thoughts" of her patient to coworkers, "Yes, I have been puking for several weeks. My owners brought me in immediately." Mockery and disdain were especially pronounced when an animal was euthanized for what had started as a preventable problem.

Occupational slang distances workers from unpleasant tasks and upsetting situations, provides a private means of communication, and is sometimes simply an exercise in creativity and wit.[30] The folks in the gastroenterology unit thought themselves particularly clever when they described their work as a specialty that "doesn't take anybody's shit" and with nicknames like "Rear Admirals" or "Guts and Butts Docs." To poke fun at some difficult clients, veterinarians call them *crocks*—medical slang for people with no apparent illness or measurable problem—who are possibly using their pets as an attention-getting measure.[31] Veterinary clients believed to be senile, unintelligent, or intoxicated may become a *CSTO* or *DSTO,* or "cat (or dog) smarter than owner."

Participation in humor creates a sense of belonging to a select inside group and often represents a transition from outsider to trusted insider.[32] My own movement from outsider researcher to acceptance in the private workspace of veterinarians, was partly accomplished through humor.[33] Participants often playfully implied that I was macabre or enjoyed being present for euthanasia procedures. Interns enjoyed mischievously asking me technical questions in front of clients so that they could later laugh at my awkward and unscientific responses. Two particularly embarrassing mishaps were told and retold at social gatherings with increasingly exaggerated detail and humorous glee. The first was a horrific accident that occurred while I was helping transport a large container packed full of animal cadavers to the crematorium. While tipping back the wheeled container to exit the elevator, I lost my balance and slipped, causing the container to tip over on top of me. The story of lifeless animals falling on my face always elicited a hearty laugh.

The second comedic event was a devilishly planned practical joke in which I was asked to manually feel inside the rectum of a bullmastiff for foreign objects. The patient had rendered himself unable to defecate by consuming an unsupervised birthday cake decorated with pieces from a Civil War chess set. I stuck my fingers into his rectum and managed to grab hold of a missing rook, which helped the patient release a gush of black diarrhea all over my face and clothes. Having anticipated this explosion, the entire clinic erupted in laughter. Undoubtedly, participating in playful repartee and good-humored teasing not only helped participants become more comfortable with me but also eased my acceptance into their world.

Language that began as taboo to novice interns later became ordinary. One intern remembered his early experiences with backstage rhetoric: "Thinking back to my first day on the job, I was disturbed by everyone so nonchalantly saying, 'We need a bag and tag.' But I guess after awhile you just sort of get used to it; I mean, that is what you're doing." In their study of human-medicine students, Allen Smith and Sherryl Kleinman show that for novices or students "joking about patients and procedures means sharing something special with the faculty, becoming a colleague."[34] Some interns eagerly took up the darker expressions of the battle-worn veterans to prove they had what it took to be a real veterinarian.

Humor allows workers who are asked to perform duties most outsiders would consider horrific to feel that it was just another day on the job. The use of humor is well documented as a tool to distance professionals from roles marked by tension, ambiguity, anxiety, frustration, uncertainty, and tragedy.[35] The majority of veterinary humor, slang, and backstage talk centers on death and euthanasia, topics characterized by high levels of tension, ambiguity, frustration, and anxiety. Plenty of professionals use dark humor to manage emotions associated with death-related experiences; medical students laugh about cadavers,[36] police officers make humorous comments about murder victims,[37] paramedics snicker at people who are beheaded in accidents,[38] anesthetists make light of mistakes that have killed patients,[39] and physicians even joke about death in the neonatal unit.[40]

At times, veterinarians ostentatiously or comically flout death by making macabre jokes about it. When an intern inquired as to how much sedative to give a dog she is preparing for euthanasia, a resident jokingly responded, "You don't need to titrate a dose, . . . because what is the worst thing that can really happen? You might kill him?" On a busy night in the critical care ward, workers may darkly joke, "I need to admit this dog, but we are pretty much out of cage space. Is there anyone looking bad enough to euthanize?" Sometimes jokes were made about killing healthy patients to ease the burden on staff: "Oh, little Fluffy has a hangnail. Have you considered euthanasia?"

Anecdotes of outrageous life-and-death negotiations with "crazy" clients and euthanasia gone amiss became a favorite topic among interns and residents. One intern, particularly known for his ability to capture even the most serious experience with raucous hilarity, told of having to listen to a client's stories about the animal for over two hours posteuthanasia. At the end of their internships, interns participated in a traditional mock award ceremony. Interns could receive awards for the longest, shortest, most bizarre, saddest, or funniest euthanasia. Awards were given to interns who made the biggest mistake, had the most euthanasia procedures in one day, and went the longest stretch without euthanizing an animal. Although many of these incidents could easily be upsetting or embarrassing, interns framed the situation as worthy of a badge of honor by making them jokes.[41]

Like physicians, veterinarians use humor to deal with feeling hopeless and frustrated over patients not expected to recover, especially when required to artificially prolong life.[42] Veterinarians are frustrated with clients who demand they prolong patients' lives beyond the possibility of recovery. As discussed in the Introduction, frustrated participants wryly joked about euthanizing such patients: "I have a cure for this dog. It is a blue solution right over here. I should just slip it in the catheter. I could just trip with a needle of blue juice and fall into him, but I can't. [*Laughs.*] I shouldn't joke like that, but there are just some where you are just that frustrated so we joke about it."

Jokes are often used to display irritation at owners who request euthanasia for their animals for reasons that seem trivial to the veterinarian. For example, participants often joked about clients who euthanized for financial reasons: "Well, if you sold half the jewelry that you have on right now, you would have more than enough to pay for things that are needed for your pet." In another example, one participant expressed frustration over being asked to euthanize an older but otherwise healthy cat because the owner wanted to move closer to her boyfriend and the only apartment she could afford did not allow pets. Her colleague jokingly responded, "I say get rid of the boyfriend instead," and the room erupted in laughter.

If it is not clear in the tone of their joking, veterinarians often felt anger, sadness, and frustration toward the pet owner in these distressing life-and-death situations. Yet they rarely displayed these emotions in front of clients. Euthanasia required substantial emotional labor from veterinarians,[43] meaning they had to suppress their own anger, sadness, and frustration to maintain desired impressions for clients. From prostitutes[44] to physicians,[45] workers commonly use humor to control, shape, and manage their feelings to create desired impressions for others. Instead of being rude or hostile to clients, out of their presence veterinarians use humor to criticize those who create stress: "If we couldn't laugh about it, we would yell at clients." Humor, slang, and laughter diffuse tensions and deflect feelings that are incompatible with the emotions (e.g., compassion and sympathy) expected of veterinary professionals.

Humor is an important tool for creating distance from emotionally troubling activities, and it helps workers feel better about distressing aspects of the job. Humor proves a socially and professionally acceptable outlet to share emotions that would otherwise make us feel vulnerable and break down emotionally. Without our having to confess weakness, humor is a safe way to acknowledge a problem and discuss serious issues.[46] Although participants spoke with trusted colleagues if they were feeling sad or depressed over a case, using humor helped them feel less of a burden on equally stressed colleagues. Rather than reacting with self-pity or sadness, participants used humor as a playful way to respond to troubling cases. Moreover, playful joking often turned into brainstorming sessions where multiple veterinarians and staff members worked together to find practical solutions for colleagues dealing with troubling cases.

Relying on Uncertainty

A patient's response to treatment is never entirely predictable: "So many things can go wrong, like you have an animal [that] comes in for trauma, and everything else is fine, but the next day it is in kidney failure because it was in shock for too long. It can be things that you can never predict. As you practice you get more and more comfortable with uncertainty." On the other hand, participants could all recall a time when overconfidence led them astray in a medical outcome. For example, many recall encouraging a client to pay for expensive treatment because the patient's outcome seemed assured, but the animal died. Like their medical counterparts,[47] veterinary students are taught the importance of balancing uncertainty with certainty because too much doubt, just as much as overconfidence, can compromise their patients' outcomes.

As an emotionally defensive tactic, relying on uncertainty includes realizing that one cannot affect certain events and resigning oneself accordingly. For example, Dr. Edwards relied on the uncertainty of patient response to treatment to ease her discomfort with euthanasia:

> I thought this dog had a shot, and I didn't want to euthanize her, . . . but let me also assure you that each individual is different. Unfortunately, this dog may never leave the hospital, and he could die in the next few days or the next few weeks, or he could live for more than a year and we just don't know. I feel okay with this euthanasia *because* we just don't know, and she could die tomorrow anyway.

Without a proper diagnosis of a terminal condition, it can be difficult for the veterinarian to agree to euthanasia. However, as Dr. Logan explained, veterinarians might rely on an uncertain outcome to justify the euthanasia:

> The cat is still urinating blood, and you think it might be cancer of the bladder, and all you want is a $300 ultrasound, and they don't

want to do it. . . . If they want to euthanize, it is most likely something bad 'cause you got far enough to establish that. You can feel okay about the euthanasia because you really can't guarantee the animal would even pull through the treatment.

By narrowing the potential diagnosis to a limited number of serious conditions, Dr. Logan embraced uncertainty to feel better about euthanizing her patient: "You can give them [clients] the justification for euthanasia because . . . they may spend all this money trying to treat something serious and the animal ends up dead anyway."

Veterinarians also embrace uncertainty when performing life-saving procedures on animals they have little faith will recover. In these cases, the pet owner insists the veterinarian do everything possible to save the animal, but participants loathe putting their patient through painful procedures on a doubtful outcome. However, veterinarians relied on uncertainty to feel better about the intervention by thinking of their patients who should have died by all medical indications but survived and are doing well. Participants often shared stories with each other of unexpected deaths from benign conditions and unlikely recoveries from serious illness. These stories reinforce the unpredictability inherent in medicine and help colleagues rely on uncertainty when struggling with difficult cases.

Creating Moral Limits

To reduce the moral ambiguity inherent in some life-and-death situations, veterinarians create moral limits to bound their behavior. Like young legal professionals, veterinarians make their ethically questionable behavior seem less so by comparing their situation to tales of extremely unethical behavior told to them in school.[48] For example, one veterinarian excused her ethically troubling actions by recalling a story about a client who asked to have her dog euthanized because it no longer matched the color scheme of her house: "I may euthanize for some iffy behavior reasons, but I would *never* euthanize because my client bought a white couch and her dog's fur is black." Many participants used tales of extremely callous owners who wished to have their animals euthanized for frivolous reasons such as the animal's breed being no longer fashionable. In reality these extreme requests rarely occur, but they are reference points and moral limits in the mind of veterinarians.

Veterinarians also made their own ethically questionable behavior seem less questionable by comparing their behavior to that of colleagues whose behavior was extreme. For example, veterinarians can gain a reputation for euthanizing too many patients: "We will nickname them 'Dr. Death' because so many of their patients are euthanized. . . . The reason may be because the vet is too lazy to try and talk clients into trying alternatives." On the other hand, a veterinarian may earn a reputation for treating animals beyond what other staff members believe reasonable: "Sometimes they don't know when to stop offering things to clients or they just want money." By characterizing the behavior of certain peers as greedy or lazy, participants relied on these moral limits to justify their own ethically questionable behavior. For example, upset that her clients wished to euthanize too early, a veterinarian eased her guilt by saying, "At least I gave her a good shot. . . . Dr. Death would have convinced the owners to euthanize a long time ago."

Finally, participants eased their discomfort with ethical uncertainty associated with euthanasia by comparing their work to other subspecialty veterinarians and animal shelter workers. As small-animal veterinarians, participants distinguished their work as less ethically challenging than other subspecialties:

> I could never be a large-animal vet or a vet involved in animal research. . . . Some things we do make me uncomfortable, but it is not as bad as what they have to do. They don't really have patients. They are just somebody's property. If the animal's economic value is low, then you can't [*uses a sarcastic tone*] *waste* money on things like anesthesia. There's a *big* difference in what we do and what they have to do. That would suck.

Veterinarians also drew sharp ethical lines between their work and the work of shelter employees. Though participants nearly universally respected the efforts of shelter workers, they also clearly held almost hostile feelings about the practice of euthanasia in animal shelters:

> I would not wish the shelter job on anyone. I think that they have a shitty job, and how they go home at night and feel comfortable with themselves I don't know. That is on them. I am not in that part of the field, and I don't choose to be. In a sense they are helping these animals technically, but I am more in the medical field, and my wish for these animals is to be healthy and to live and to find homes and to be medically treated.

By defining the actions of shelter workers and fellow veterinarians as morally questionable, participants shaped their actions as valid and eased their discomfort with the ethical uncertainty they faced in their own work.

Using the Owner

Veterinarians relieve emotional discomfort related to euthanasia dilemmas by both blaming and sympathizing with clients.[49] Participants blamed clients for their moral dilemma when clients prolonged a suffering animal's life by asking the veterinarian to keep it alive through medical intervention. In these cases veterinarians may prefer to euthanize, but they feel as though their hands are tied by delusional, manipulative, or unrealistic owners:

> I want to fix what is treatable where the chance is realistic, . . . but when there is a really grave prognosis, . . . sometimes I really hate it when owners decide to treat. I will lay it all out for them and give them all the information and the prognosis and everything, but [if] they are like, "Well, I really have to give him a chance," who am I to say no? It is really their decision.

While sustaining the life of some animals causes a great deal of moral stress for the veterinarian, blaming clients creates emotional distance to help the veterinarian get the job done.

On the other hand, veterinarians were sympathetic to clients who were strongly bonded to their animals and recognized that clients need not be crazy or unrealistic to be reluctant to permit euthanasia.[50] Participants developed strong bonds of their own with patients and described losing touch with reality such that they no longer set reasonable limits on procedures designed to extend the life of patients. Veterinarians occasionally have difficulty accepting that a patient's physical problems can no longer be controlled and, as a result, have a tough time establishing limitations on end-of-life care. Thus, they were often sympathetic to clients in this situation.

Most often participants blamed pet owners to ease their discomfort with killing animals. If clients had not taken basic precautions to prevent the animal's grim situation, veterinarians held them responsible for the animal's death. Dr. Black expressed her anger with her clients for not vaccinating their dog who was later attacked by a stray dog suspected of having rabies:

> The people were so stupid, and it was their own stupidity that caused this whole, entire problem. . . . I am sitting there talking to them about euthanizing their healthy Chihuahua with a broken leg and a bite wound because they had never vaccinated her for rabies. . . . It got euthanized because they are stupid. It was their fault, and it sucks that the animal has to suffer for it.

Notice that, although Dr. Black euthanized the animal herself, it is clear that she used her client to distance herself from the act when she said, "It got euthanized." Some pet owners allowed benign medical problems to become life threatening before seeking treatment. If the owner appeared indifferent to obvious suffering, culpability was easily assigned to the client. For example, after euthanizing a dog with a severe, foul-smelling skin condition that had been festering for months, Dr. Hill clearly held the client responsible for the death of the animal: "Neglect like this is always disgusting, but it is a lot worse when I have to kill them *because* the owner let it get out of hand and now there is not a lot we can do for them. That is really criminal."

Pet owners could be blameworthy if they were not interested in spending reasonable amounts or making some effort to avoid euthanasia. These clients angered Dr. Miller: "Often I am trying to finagle so we can treat this poor pet, and they are like, 'No, I don't really want to spend a dime.' I want to beat them, especially if they drive away in a Mercedes, and then I just really want to fucking kill them." Of course, standards for minimal efforts and reasonable amounts expected of pet owners varied from veterinarian to veterinarian. However, when those standards were not met, veterinarians often lessened their feelings of sadness or guilt over the death of the patient by blaming pet owners: "The one thing I have learned is that I shouldn't feel guilty about euthanizing animals when their owners suck and don't care about their animals."

These statements clearly show that clients labeled bad owners are not considered especially deserving of the veterinarian's sympathy. While most participants tried to hide their emotions from clients, some subtly chastised them. Others, like Dr. Smith, felt better when they openly advocated for patients by giving their clients a hard time:

> If it is solely a financial thing, I don't ever want anyone to leave feeling like they did the right thing and it wasn't. I will make this really clear to them that this is a financial decision but that there are things we can do and the animal would do just fine with treatment. . . . I am going to give them a hard time so that I feel better that I gave it a shot to save the animal.

Like shelter workers who sometimes try to instill guilt in those who surrender their animals,[51] some veterinarians did the same to "bad" owners. However, educating bad clients to make them better future pet owners also provided veterinarians some relief after the euthanasia: "Whenever I euthanize for aggressive behavior and I think the owners did something to encourage it,

I try to educate them . . . so the person may want to think about how they treat their next dog." By focusing on educating owners, the veterinarian could think about helping animals in general rather than saving one specific patient.

When euthanasia felt dirty, or less than legitimate, veterinarians tried to forget their anger at bad clients by focusing on those pet owners who did the utmost for their animals. For example, frustrated with one owner's lack of commitment to a pet, the veterinarian redirected her focus: "I try to think about all those owners who really go the distance for their animals." Dr. Miller was clearly inspired when impoverished pet owners went to extraordinary lengths to raise the necessary funds to pay for treatment:

> They will say, "I can get you $25 this week," and you know that is really what they can get you. It hits home to what a sacrifice it is that they are willing to spend $2,000 to get their dog's surgery. You would be paying this for a year, like every spare dollar that you have would go toward this pet. This is the extra slap in the face when you have this [other] person drive off in a Mercedes who wasn't willing to do the same surgery. That is really touching.

Participants relied on this strategy so much that nearly early every time I asked them to tell me about an occasion an owner frustrated them they also mention a time when clients surpassed their expectations: "You have owners who throw out animals like trash, but you also have these people who you think don't have any money but will do all this amazing shit for their animal." Sympathetic to clients who appeared to have strong bonds with their animals, veterinarians used these pet owners to feel better and forget about clients who seemed less attached to their animals.

In addition to blaming clients, participants sometimes used the client to ease their discomfort with euthanasia by sympathizing with the client; focusing on the hurdles, difficulties, and complexities for clients. For example, although he hoped his clients would choose surgery over euthanasia, when they did not Dr. Stevens focused on their potential economic liability:

> Some people will destroy their life doing surgery on an animal. You will destroy their life. The surgery will cost $4,000, and it would save the cat's life, but $4,000 to some people is a huge deal. Yes, there is CareCredit, but it is still a credit card, . . . and if they are late one payment, 25 percent interest gets tacked on. . . . If they are late and we put them to collections, they will never buy a car. They will never buy a house. They will never be able to get their life completely in

order because of a dog or a cat. I hate to say that as a vet, and that is awful to say that as a vet, but at the same time, I don't want to ruin anybody's life.

By focusing on how financing the animal's treatment could negatively influence the owner's life, participants could alleviate their own discomfort over euthanizing patients.

Veterinarians sometimes used the pet owner to shift their discomfort with the rationale for euthanasia toward relieving the stress of distraught clients. For example, Dr. Buford euthanized two healthy pit bulls because she sympathized with her client, who was unable to find a home for them and could not afford to keep them. The client did not want to take them to a shelter because she thought they would be euthanized because of their breed and could not bear the thought of them dying alone in a shelter with strangers. Dr. Buford explained, "I think it was her reaction that really made me kind of okay with it. I felt like she was looking at me as her last resort. Rather than have this pregnant lady be so stressed and upset for these dogs that she loved, I just did it." Although this was a situation that the veterinarian would normally challenge, she agreed to the euthanasia without much resistance for the sake of the client's feelings.

Using the Animal

When they were asked to sustain the life of animals they would rather euthanize or to euthanize animals they would rather not, veterinarians made themselves feel better by doing their best to ensure the animal's comfort. Although Dr. Green described feeling like a monster for treating some patients, she found comfort in empathizing with patients and doing her best to ensure their comfort:

> The ones you really hate the most are the really critical ones, where clients want us to do everything and they [the animals] are suffering. . . . You can feel like a real *monster* keeping them alive sometimes. . . . You have to do everything to make them feel comfortable. It is hard, but I try to comfort myself with the fact that . . . I am doing everything I can to make them comfortable short of euthanizing them, so I don't feel like I am a monster.

To deal with the prospect of euthanizing animals, participants, like shelter workers,[52] also eased their discomfort by doing their best to make the euthanasia process as comfortable as possible for the animal. Arnold Arluke's shelter workers made special efforts to concentrate on becoming technically proficient at the methodology of killing and "tried to make this experience as 'good' as possible for the animals and, in so doing, felt better themselves."[53]

For many participants, comforting and empathizing with the animal meant having the pet owner present for the animal's benefit. Although the client's presence adds additional stress for the veterinarian, most believe that the animal is more comfortable and relaxed around familiar faces. If the owner was unable or did not wish to be present for the euthanasia, participants would often find the patient's favorite technician to assist—with the hope of helping the animal feel less anxious. To make patients happy and relaxed, participants especially enjoyed feeding animals treats or giving them a special meal of their favorite foods. Some veterinarians liked to spend time with the animal or take them for a final walk outside. Regardless of where the euthanasia took place, participants did their best to make it a less distressing environment. Veterinarians tranquilized the animals to help them relax[54] and often offered gentle touches during the euthanasia: "We love to give tummy scratches or a head rub."

In sympathizing with the animal and making the experience comfortable, Arluke argues that shelter workers were able to selectively focus "on the technique of killing—and not on why it needed to be done or how they felt about doing it."[55] Like other occupational groups, such as shelter workers[56] and nurses,[57] veterinarians drew attention away from conflicting feelings or dirty aspects of their work by focusing on caring for the needs of patients. Some practices intended to ease the animal's anxiety arguably served more to relieve the veterinarian's tension and stress. For example, Dr. Turner described how she talks to her patients as she euthanizes them when the pet owners are not present:

> Like with cats it's more of a soothing voice, and with dogs I will walk in and reassure them and say, "Oh, Frankie, you're such a good boy, aren' you? You've been such a good boy. Do you know how much we love you, Frankie? And your mommy and daddy love you, and they are so sorry that they can't be here. And they just want me to tell you what a good boy you are." We know they don't understand, but it actually *makes us feel better*. (Emphasis added)

By easing the animal's stress with a comforting tone of voice, veterinarians admittedly not only help patients die "peacefully" but also help themselves cope with the stress of killing.

Like shelter workers,[58] veterinarians also used the animal by focusing on the animal's welfare to help justify euthanasia. In other words, participants found the death of certain animals an appropriate means to end suffering: "Those animals that sit in the ICU that have zero prognosis of recovering and they feel horrible—those kinds of euthanasias should not make you feel bad, but you should feel good." Although the deaths of animals in immediate discomfort were easiest to justify, veterinarians also rationalized euthanasia as a tool to *prevent* suffering. In the case of a terminal illness, for example, veterinarians sometimes justified euthanizing the patient earlier than they would have preferred by viewing it as preventing suffering in the patient's future. For some animals it was better than the alternative, spending the rest of their lives in an overcrowded animal shelter.

Veterinarians sometimes coped with euthanasia by viewing it as a better alternative to a life of starving or dying a painful death. I was told at least one horror story in nearly every hospital I visited of uncaring and neglectful pet owners who abandoned their animal out in the country or on the side of the highway. While the exact details of how the fate of the animals became known to staff varied, the news of the animals' tragic deaths somehow made its way to the hospital, leaving the veterinarians guilt ridden for having refused to euthanize the animals. Some stories involved the client euthanizing the animal at home by less humane methods. In one especially gruesome such story, the client was so angered at the veterinarian's refusal to euthanize that he brutally killed the animal in the hospital's parking lot and left the body as revenge. Regardless of the authenticity of these events, the telling of such tales reveals a common fear among veterinarians that patients might suffer if veterinarians refuse an owner's request for euthanasia. Participants eased their ethical discomfort with some euthanasia procedures by viewing them as a better alternative for the animal than abandonment or painful death.

Accentuating the Positive: Euthanasia as Rewarding

Veterinarians dislike using every treatment available for patients when cure—or even comfort—is not in the cards. Thus, because they have the legal ability to end their patients' suffering, many in veterinary medicine see euthanasia as a luxury available to them—one with a lot of difficult ethical dilemmas, but a privilege nonetheless. Familiar with the anguish of doing everything possible to sustain the lives of suffering patients, participants frequently expressed sympathy for their medical counterparts: "A lot of my friends are MDs and you hear them tell stories that they were forced to anesthetize this ninety-year-old woman with Alzheimer's to do a total hip. I was like that is horrible. They just describe a horrible quality of life for many of their patients."

Despite all the potential problems and stresses the option of euthanasia brings to the practice of veterinary medicine, nearly all participants strongly believed that euthanasia was positive for the profession: "I definitely think that it is something that veterinary medicine has that is great in terms of being able to end suffering and to not have to watch . . . quality of life go in a downward spiral. . . . I think doctors have to see a lot of [that] in human medicine." Understanding that euthanasia in human medicine would come with its own set of ethical dilemmas for medical practitioners, some participants pondered what it would be like to practice human medicine without euthanasia as a legal option. One veterinarian said, "Although I know they experience pain, my patients can't speak. . . . I couldn't imagine what it would be like for someone to beg and plead with me to end their suffering and it not be legal to help them—I would feel so helpless."

Time and time again, veterinarians described euthanasia as both the best and worst part of their job. Although most participants were quick to illustrate the ways euthanasia is fraught with dilemmas and can feel distasteful, they simultaneously depict it as a tremendously rewarding and gratifying part of their work. In fact, when the goal of euthanasia is to end the pain and suffering of animals, veterinarians, like shelter workers,[59] often report an overwhelming sense of relief after performing euthanasia. Noting the potentially heroic feelings euthanasia can provoke, Dr. Logan summed up a common sentiment: "If you have watched your patient suffer for weeks and . . . you finally convince them [the clients] to euthanize, it is an even better feeling—it is a really good feeling." Thus, the definition of professional success for these veterinarians includes both healing animals and ending their suffering through euthanasia.

In the beginning of their internships, interns fairly exclusively defined *success* as solving a difficult diagnosis or saving the life of an injured patient. The cases that ended in euthanasia always seemed failures. However, as time went on, novices began to broaden their definition of success to include euthanasia, which could be especially rewarding for interns who felt underappreciated by staff and supervisors:

During the times in the internship when I hadn't really had much in the way of encouragement, helping owners emotionally can be wonderfully rewarding. You know your follow-up is not that great, and you are still dashing around all crazy, and you are unsure, and

you don't know as much, and you make mistakes. There are a lot of
negative criticisms [from supervisors] that flow around here, and it is
nice to hear something positive. Sometimes . . . the only thanks or
encouragement you get is with euthanasia. The clients will send you
cards and thank-you letters for killing their animals a lot faster than
they will for saving their animal. Those thank-you cards and the ap-
preciation are nice to hear when you feel like you do nothing right.
The client is just so grateful that you helped them through such a
difficult time that they give you a lot in return.

Many interns also found helping clients emotionally during euthanasia to be
a very rewarding aspect of their job. Dr. Green explained, "Being there for
the euthanasia of someone's animal is an experience that a lot of people don't
have access to—about how people think and feel about their animals. . . . It
is like I get a private screening to very intimate times for people that a lot of
other people never get to experience."

For many veterinarians, having empathy and, more importantly, the ability to convey it effectively to clients is a key part of their definition of what
it means to be a good and competent veterinarian. As seen in Chapter 3,
veterinarians help clients manage emotions related to pet loss and euthanasia.
For many participants the ability to help clients during the stressful time of
pet loss is part of what attracted them to the profession in the first place: "I
don't mind the intimate, emotional part of it. . . . I think helping owners
emotionally is an important part of veterinary medicine. Good euthanasia
can be as rewarding as healing animals." In a similar way, abortion counselors
"spoke with immense satisfaction of . . . really 'being there' for the woman
and helping her make it through a difficult time."[60] Thus, as scholars suggest,
veterinarians perform emotion work to not only meet job requirements but
also shape a positive identity and fulfill important commitments to self.[61]
For many participants veterinarians who are more caring and sensitive to the
anxieties and emotional needs of clients are better veterinarians.

Ritualizing

Workers charged with emotionally difficult tasks develop rituals to get the job
done, but the routines also provide them comfort.[62] In fact, scholars suggest
that having a ritual or ceremony marking the occasion can provide comfort
for those grieving the loss of a pet.[63] As discussed in Chapter 2, "Creating
a Good Death," veterinarians have created informal routines that not only
ease the burden of their work but also enhance the experience for the animal

patient and human client. One of these is the client's presence during the death of the animal, which most participants believed was important for the patient as well as the owner.

Although euthanasia can be deeply rewarding and satisfying for the veterinarian, it loses its sacredness when the owners do not participate. For example, early in one of our interviews, Dr. Fury tried his best to convince me that he cared about the pet owners' presence only for the sake of the patient; however, in a later interview he began to cry as he admitted their presence was also an important emotional support for him:

> The pet being stroked and petted and being spoken to—for [the pet] and me [that] is so much more worth it, just having the comfort of [the owners] saying good-bye. I feel like owners owe it to their pets— I mean, animals are great. They'll just give you their heart unconditionally. That type of devotion—you need to be able to stand up and take their death. [*Sobbing.*] And I do feel better when people decide to stay. . . . If you don't stay . . . the animal is taken into the back, and that's it. How can that be the end of such a meaningful relationship?

Like Dr. Fury, several participants cried or held back tears when discussing nonwitness euthanasia. In many of my interviews with participants, the topic was the most emotionally upsetting part of the interview. The ritual for euthanizing an animal without clients present that nearly every veterinarian had was often not as meaningful to the veterinarian as the one with clients present. Although having the client present at the euthanasia often made it more time consuming, nearly all participants strongly preferred to euthanize patients with their owners present.

Although many participants took pride in their ability to stage a meaningful euthanasia experience for patients and their owners, they sometimes dismissed its benefits for themselves. As implied in Temple Grandin's concept of sacred ritual, the performance aspects of killing an animal can be psychologically important for workers.[64] Most participants' rituals often mirrored Grandin's suggestion to create a calming atmosphere for the animal, but only a few followed her suggestion of some additional act of reverence such as bowing one's head or a moment of silence for the benefit of the worker. One participant's ritual, rarely used by others, included saying the following after each euthanasia procedure: "I am reminded of the value of life and the decision to sacrifice life so that priorities of my culture are realized. I understand my role in the loss of the life; I will not ignore this sacrifice, and I am grateful for the benefits that come at this cost."

Other Strategies

In addition to the tension- and emotion-management techniques outlined in the preceding, participants used other strategies. Some participants relied heavily on social support from friends and family, but most were uncomfortable talking to outsiders, who may not understand their dilemmas. A small proportion of participants sought assistance from mental health professionals to deal with emotions associated with euthanasia in their work, among other issues. Although professionals have long been advocates of pet-loss support groups for veterinarians,[65] they are rare. However, some clinics regularly address emotionally upsetting issues in scheduled support meetings.[66] Though a few participants turned to negative coping mechanisms such as alcohol consumption or drug use to alleviate euthanasia-related stress, others relied on strategies such as regular exercise, healthy eating habits, regular vacations, hobbies, "expressive writing,"[67] and enjoying the times they were off work. As shelter workers also report,[68] many participants felt better after a difficult euthanasia by going home after work and giving extra attention to their animals.

Failed Emotion Management

To avoid euthanasia-related stress, veterinary professionals rely on the problem-focused strategies outlined in Chapter 1 and the emotion-focused strategies outlined earlier, including emotional distancing techniques, relying on uncertainty, creating moral limits, using the owner, using the animal, accentuating the positive, and ritualizing. While some of the problem-focused and emotion-focused techniques were, at first, problematic for novice interns, by the end of their internship most adopted several that they would refine over time. However, even the strategies of veterinarians with many years of experience were far from perfect. For example, nearly all participants occasionally were preoccupied by certain cases and needed to reminisce or talk about the circumstances of the case. Veterinarians commonly report at least some uneasiness over certain aspects of euthanasia in their work.[69] Participants reported varying levels of sadness, grief, frustration, guilt, anxiety, anger, irritability, resentment, and remorse.

The ways veterinarians coped with stress changed over time as they continually reassessed and refined their techniques.[70] At times, as predicted in the coping literature, some participants overly relied on emotion-focused strategies for solvable problems.[71] For a few of these participants the use of emotion-focused tactics became almost pathological, as potentially solvable problems were regularly laughed off or dismissed as inevitable parts of the job. Under pressure from colleagues or supervisors to conform to hospital norms, some participants gave in to peer pressure and then relied on emotion-focused strategies to ease their discomfort. Young interns, for example, often under nearly around-the-clock pressure, were especially vulnerable: "[When it came to a difficult case and there was disagreement], it was a lot easier to euthanize than it [was] to work it up." Exclusive focus on emotion-based coping has the potential to draw attention away from the broader structures and organizational policies that contribute to and maintain the stress-inducing situation. In this case the traditional practice of having interns work extraordinarily long hours, leading to negative-coping situations, remains unquestioned.

Euthanasia of healthy animals with no behavioral or health problems is a major source of job dissatisfaction for veterinarians, as it is for shelter workers and animal control officers.[72] Euthanizing animals that were simply unwanted by their owners was the most problematic for nearly all participants, and for some, it threatened their identity: "When I do those, I feel less like a doctor and more like a shelter worker." Participants also reported considerable stress over clients who refused to let go of sick animals: "Watching a patient suffer is one of the most depressing parts of my job. . . . People want to keep them on a ventilator, and I have to watch them suffer." For some veterinarians it was torture to even look at these patients: "It can get so bad that nobody wants to look at the animal during rounds. . . . We talk about the case but stare anywhere but that cage. It is terrible."

One of the most difficult euthanasia procedures for almost every participant was euthanizing an animal to whom they had developed an attachment. Despite every novice learning mechanisms to distance him- or herself emotionally—almost as a rite of passage—most became attached to a particular patient such that they were upset and distraught upon its death. Even veterinarians with years of experience had varying successes and failures with emotional distance as a coping mechanism. Attachments could become quite strong in a relatively short time but were especially strong when the veterinarian helped an animal battle an illness over the course of several weeks, months, or even years. Research confirms that the higher the degree of attachment, the greater the emotional difficulty.[73]

Distancing techniques, helpful for managing problematic emotions in difficult situations, are not without a potential dark side. For example, veterinarian Cydria Manette expresses concern that, "by distancing ourselves from . . . our feelings, we remove ourselves from experiencing not only fear and guilt, but also empathy and compassion."[74] In other words, the techniques that operate to create emotional distance from troubling experiences may also distance professionals from those they are charged with helping such that they become callous, jaded, or detached. This could also lead to practitioners categorically resenting patients and clients, and adversarial veterinarian-client or veterinarian-patient relationships. Thus, emotional distancing techniques have the potential to become maladaptive coping strategies with dysfunctional outcomes.

Many occupational groups that deal with death and dying argue that emotional distancing techniques such as gallows humor are important for surviving in the job. The use of language that disparages and depersonalizes death lessens the psychological impact on workers. Phrases to describe euthanasia such as "given the blue juice," "sent to doggie heaven," "sent paws up," or "put to sleep" distance the act of killing by sanitizing it in euphemism—even if the euphemisms are dark or comedic. However, for some, colleagues using this tactic were showing signs of burnout or too much disconnect: "I thought there was a problem when he would refer to euthanasia—he used the term *nuke*, like 'I need to go nuke this dog.' It made me sick every time he would say those words." Once a person becomes jaded, using these techniques can exacerbate anger, cynicism, and impatience.

Admitting that distancing techniques can be a precarious balancing act, most veterinarians defend their use: "It is not that we don't have respect for the situation, and it is not that we are not sad about the situation; . . . we have all these emotions that we have to deal with in some way." Most participants staunchly defended the use of humor as essential for survival in their jobs: "If we can't laugh about it, we would cry all the time." Practitioners who could not find a balance between detachment and concern in either direction found clinical work unbearably stressful, tiresome, and unrewarding. To remedy this situation, most veterinarians learned to balance the seemingly incongruent feelings: "You can reconcile the fact that you may experience a certain humor about the death of your patients with the fact that you really care. Over time that doesn't seem like a contradiction to you; . . . you know that you care, and you know that you use humor to survive . . . because we really do *care* deeply about our patients."

In my experience among veterinarians, emotionally distancing techniques were not incompatible with concern for colleagues, clients, or patients. For the most part, techniques such as humor, slang, and laughter neutralized emotionally tense situations, making difficult situations bearable. Despite the use of such distancing techniques, most practitioners were able to continue to care and feel connected to their work. Most participants carefully controlled their detachment from clients and patients because it seemed antithetical to their sense of themselves as animal-loving, caring, and compassionate people.

Although some participants could be considered rude surgeons or arrogant residents who seemed to have tipped the delicate balance, most were compassionate and sensitive doctors with impressive empathy for their clients and patients.

Relying on the uncertainty of clinical medicine to manage their discomfort with euthanasia was an effective strategy for some participants. Uncertainty made others feel worse. For example, some veterinarians could find comfort in euthanizing animals they would rather not by resigning themselves to the fact that the outcome is never certain and the animal could experience painful surgery only to die in the end. But others focused on the chance that the animal would beat the odds and recover if only given the chance. Like human-medicine personnel, veterinarians sometimes struggle with deaths of patients that involve opposing opinions among clinicians[75] and diagnostic and prognostic uncertainty.[76]

Euthanizing large numbers of animals was troublesome for nearly every participant, and most recalled specific times when they felt overwhelmed by the number of animals they euthanized. One intern even changed her intended specialty from emergency and critical care (a specialty known to deal a lot with euthanasia) to pathology—where she could avoid euthanasia because her patients would already be dead. Another participant noted that her chosen field of ophthalmology "has the added benefit of rarely having to euthanize patients." A heavy death toll is clearly associated with greater degree of worker distress among shelter workers, and not surprisingly, veterinarians also had difficulty with it.[77]

Several participants noted a particular characteristic of a patient or a client that was always upsetting for them. For example, euthanizing young animals was distressing for almost every participant as was euthanizing animals that resembled the veterinarian's own companion animals. This might mean a particular species of animal, breed, coat color, or other similarity to their own companions. For example, one veterinarian had a weakness for a specific dog breed: "I certainly have a trigger for German shepherds 'cause I have a German shepherd. . . . It will sort of pull at my heartstrings when I'm euthanizing a German shepherd." Others struggled when they identified with the client: "It is hard, especially if they are young women too. If I can identify with them or if it is a young woman euthanizing a cat and she is alone, I pretty much cry before it starts." Both male and female veterinarians admitted discomfort at witnessing male clients cry: "Usually the more blue collar and rough the guy is, the harder it is." Some had emotional difficulty euthanizing elderly people's animals, and for others, having children in the room made a euthanasia procedure more difficult.

Participants had difficulty euthanizing patients when their clients seem indifferent to the loss of the pet: "It offends me the most when they seem to have a lack of caring. My total pet peeve frustration is when I feel like quite obviously I care more about their pet than they do." For some veterinarians, like Dr. Spencer, what makes a good euthanasia or a bad euthanasia is whether the owner is upset:

> If they're not upset, then that sucks. Not that I want to see them upset, but it's hard to watch something die and have no one care. . . . If they're not really upset when it happens, you can think it wasn't a difficult decision for them to make. And how can that decision not be difficult? . . . But for some people it's not. . . . The only real reason to euthanize is because you love them enough to euthanize them. But if that's clearly not the case, then it makes euthanizing . . . feel sort of dirty. . . . It is much harder for me when owners don't care or I think they don't care. Those just feel icky, like taking out the trash or something.

When pet owners did not seem attached to their animal, euthanasia was an unpleasant job, akin to taking out the trash. However, these cases contrasted with the ones that gave many participants joy:

> Euthanasia can be a nice reminder of how special animals can be to people. . . . I really love it when I have, like, seventeen-year-old boys crying and kissing their dead dog. I think it's one of the most beautiful things that you can see. You get to see their bond really intensely— the depth of that connection. And who gets to see that? Like that, they are totally naked. They are just vulnerable. It can be a beautiful thing. It is sad, but it . . . makes you feel good too.

Although participants recognized that there were a variety of legitimate reasons that clients might choose for not being with their animals during euthanasia, euthanizing animals without the clients present was emotionally difficult for many participants. For example, even though he was upset at his clients for treating their animal as a disposable product, Dr. Logan wanted them at the euthanasia procedure: "Remember those people who wanted to move to Virginia? They said, 'Well, I want to euthanize this cat, and I will just get a new cat when I move to Virginia.' They didn't even want to be with their cat and comfort her during the euthanasia. That makes me sad." Like human-medicine personnel, veterinarians were upset by "relatives" abandoning the dying.[78] For many participants, like Dr. Davis, it was harder to feel as though they made death as comfortable as possible for the animal:

> I hate euthanizing a pet when they are in unfamiliar territory and around unfamiliar faces. I hate it. . . . You are walking down the hall, and the animal is looking back at their owner walking out the door. I hate it. That is the worst. . . . I usually cry when the owners aren't there. . . . That cat or that dog doesn't know me from anybody. I think animals know who their owners are, and it is an uncomfortable, scary situation for them to be in here anyway, and here we are killing it. It is very uncomfortable for me when they [clients] are not involved.

All told, Dr. Davis said that she hated owners not being present during euthanasia procedures approximately ten times in this interview. When asked why they would prefer owners to be present given that their presence adds significant time, most cited the calming and comfort the animal received from the owner's presence and said that it lifted the burden off them of comforting the animal.

Without the clients' presence during euthanasia, veterinarians had far more difficulty using the owner to deflect responsibility. As Dr. Turner explained, having the owners around during the procedure was especially important when the veterinarian was not completely in agreement with the rationale for euthanasia:

> It is almost like the owner is the buffer. . . . When the owner is not there, you are trying to tell the pet you are so sorry [*crying*], but it kind of falls on you. . . . I feel complicit in something. . . . Sometimes I can't look that patient in the eye and tell them I did everything that I could. It is a shitty feeling. . . . It feels much more personal to me when the owners are not there. It is one thing when the owners are not there and the patient is suffering—I feel totally comfortable with that. But in cases where it is really unfortunate and you really wish it didn't have to go this way and the owner is not there, those fucking suck.

For some participants whether the client was present made no difference in their ability to use the client to transfer responsibility: "I could just think in my head that this is their decision and they are making this call; I am just carrying out their wishes." For others, without the clients' presence, the strategy proved considerably more difficult to use, especially while performing the euthanasia procedure.

Killing an animal with an excellent prognosis primarily because of finances can feel dirty, and for some it was the worst part of their job as veterinarians. In some cases, it was easy to blame greedy clients who refused to spend money on an animal they saw as easily replaceable. This strategy did not work so well when participants loved their animals and wanted to provide the necessary medical care but did not have the funds. Dr. Deaver and other veterinarians reported feeling like a murderer in these cases:

> Those are probably the most irritating . . . because the owners don't have the money, and there are no options, and you are just fucked. That is a really frustrating situation because then on top of having to euthanize a pretty treatable animal, you are sad for the owner on top of it. They don't want to lose their pet, and they don't want to feel guilty like they are not doing the best for their pet. That is a shitty situation all around. Mostly in those situations I feel really guilty for the pet. That is when I kind of feel like a murderer.

Veterinarians accept the reality that procedures to save or prolong life may be cost prohibitive for some clients: "I would say that probably most cases have at least a small financial element to [them]—if it is not the governing factor. . . . I mean, it is just part of the veterinary profession. It doesn't stop bothering us, but we all just get used to it." Like human-medicine personnel, veterinarians were also less able to cope with deaths that involved staff shortages,[79] budget cuts, failing technologies,[80] and a lack of resources.[81] Although they get used to it, knowing that treatment is possible but out of reach because of the expense makes it all the more difficult to come to terms with euthanasia.

Veterinarians experience, as we all do, personal and work-related stressors from time to time. Specific work-related stressors noted among veterinarians include dissatisfaction with income;[82] long working hours;[83] lack of resources;[84] and poor relationships with colleagues, managers, and clients.[85] In addition to these general job stressors are the well-documented psychological ramifications of euthanasia-related work found among shelter employees,[86] veterinarians,[87] animal researchers,[88] veterinary technicians,[89] and animal control officers.[90] Euthanasia-related strain is associated with higher degrees of overall job strain, work-to-family conflict, somatic complaints (such as headaches), substance abuse, and a lower degree of job satisfaction.[91]

Despite the use of a variety of problem-focused and emotion-focused techniques to solve problems and manage emotional discomfort, veterinarians continue to experience at least some uneasiness regarding this aspect of their job. For a few participants, euthanasia-related concerns remained the worst part of their job. While the amount and kind of tension end-of-life situations provoked varied from participant to participant, nearly everyone experienced some level of distress, ranging from only slightly discernible to high levels of emotional distress. By contrast, when physical and emotional coping strategies worked, veterinarians found their work rewarding. Euthanasia may always be shrouded in ambivalence.

Conclusion

Animals as Property and Patients

From my first few days in the world of veterinary medicine until my very last day, the ambiguous social status of companion animals was visually clear to me. On any given day, in one room of an animal hospital sits a healthy two-year-old cat scheduled to be put to sleep because his owners can't afford the relatively simple procedure required to unblock his urethra and return him to good health. Across the hall sits a fourteen-year-old, blind, paralyzed dog getting thousands of dollars of surgical care and around-the-clock life-sustaining treatment in hopes of buying his owners another few months with their animal. When I made note of this situation during an interview, one of my favorite veterinarians said to me:

> It is Murphy's Law of veterinary medicine that the owner who is willing to do everything has the pet who is not fixable, and the owner who is not willing to do shit has the pet who is an easy fix. It is so frustrating! You may want to treat your pet, but your pet isn't fixable. But over here I have a two-year-old cat who can't pee. Give me a couple of days and a few hundred bucks, and we can have you a great cat, but instead both of them end up dead! It is so frustrating.

Over and over again, I am reminded of this unfortunate conundrum as veterinarians complain about the ambiguous status of the animals in their care: "You've got one person that's just throwing money at you for a problem that you can't fix and then other people that can't or won't pay for problems that you can fix."

During my last few weeks in the hospital I was shadowing a new cohort of interns and had begun to think of myself a pretty good amateur veterinarian because I "cured" a feline patient of cancer. A woman brought her cat to the hospital for euthanasia because of steadily growing stomach masses. The owner said she could not afford the diagnostic or treatment options the intern discussed with her and, after signing the necessary paperwork, left the examination room. As I had done many times before, I carried the cat to the back to help prepare her for euthanasia when I noticed that the four-year-old animal did not, in fact, have multiple tumors.

The "tumors" were balls of matted hair. When the intern examined them, she knew instantly that I was right and ran off excitedly after the owner. Finding the cat's owners getting into their car, the veterinarian said, "I have great news! It is just matted hair and not cancer, so you can take your cat home." The woman responded casually, "Oh, no. We were prepared to just let her go and not have a cat for now. Just go ahead and euthanize her." Excitement drained from the young veterinarian, and she told the owner she was not comfortable with that request. She asked the owner to come in and instead sign paperwork surrendering her cat to the care of the hospital.

Although the owner agreed to allow the intern to try to find her cat a new home, the veterinarian was left frustrated and angered by the situation:

> For somebody not to know that that was a hair mat I guess is okay. . . .
> To me, that just means that they don't really touch their cat. That is
> fine, but when they found out that it was just a hair mat, their reac-
> tion to that was really shocking to me. You saw; she just waved it off
> to me and was like, "Just kill it." I thought, "Do you even know what
> you are asking me to do? I am going to kill your cat over a hair mat?
> I don't think so!"

Throughout my time in veterinary hospitals, I had seen similar situations and knew that this young, idealistic veterinarian was going to get used to pet owners who do not seem to share the moral value she places on animals. In fact, decisions around end-of-life care and euthanasia are among the biggest ethical concerns for interns, residents, and experienced veterinarians alike as they are memorable, complex, and contain deep and unresolved tensions inherent in human-animal relationships.

Veterinarians sort out and work through life-and-death conflicts with their clients every day. And when unable to resolve disagreements with pet owners, veterinarians must make difficult ethical decisions about the animals in their care. Given the ambiguity arising from the treatment of nonhuman animals simultaneously as subjects and objects,[1] a veterinarian's valuation of an animal may differ from the client's. As veterinary ethicists might predict, participants struggled to balance their dual roles as medical provider to animals and service provider to clients.[2] Bernard Rollin considers a veterinarian's moral obligations to animals and clients to be so important to veterinary medicine that he calls it "the fundamental question of veterinary ethics."[3]

In the end-of-life disagreements between veterinarians and their clients outlined in Chapter 1, three major sources of ethical and moral tension clearly emerge: differences in values regarding the importance of animals, differences in beliefs regarding a pet owner's responsibility to pets, and differences in assessment of the interest of animals.[4] First, as in the examples earlier in this chapter, differing attitudes regarding animals caused disagreements between the veterinarian and the client. Some pet owners were willing to go into debt to save the lives of their companion animals, while others chose euthanasia because they were unwilling to spend minimal amounts on their animals. Participants also made their own distinctions between animals, dismissing some as "just a chicken" or "just a mouse" while grieving over the loss of others. Moreover, though sensitive to a budding debate over terminology regarding companion animals,[5] participants referred to animals equally and interchangeably as both "patients" receiving care and as their owner's "property." Regardless of any veterinarian's particular moral view of animals along a spectrum from subject to object, she or he is likely to encounter owners with different views and contradictory beliefs.

The second major source of veterinarian-client conflict demonstrated in Chapter 1 involves differences in beliefs regarding human responsibility to companion animals. Although legal statutes mandate provision of food, water, and shelter, ideal standards of care—beyond the minimum required by law—varied from veterinarian to veterinarian and from client to client. Veterinarians considered some clients unreasonable for choosing or not choosing certain treatment options for their animals. Every participant had a story about clients who went too far and those who did not do near enough for their pet animals. Clients also had their own ideas about the proper treatment owed to animals. For example, some people believe it is excessive or even morally wrong to provide veterinary specialties such as ophthalmology, dermatology, and oncology to nonhuman animals. Some clients even laughed out loud when veterinarians suggested they take their pet to see a cardiac specialist or to receive chemotherapy. In other words, even when veterinarians and clients are on the same page regarding the moral status of companion animals, they may still debate the level of veterinary care owed to animals.

The third major source of veterinarian-client conflict highlighted in Chapter 1 involves difference in defining the interests of animals. Even in cases where the veterinarian and the client both want to serve the best interests of the animal they may disagree on what is best for the animal. Sometimes these disagreements are easily dispatched when the veterinarian educates the client. However, the situation becomes even more complicated when veterinary experts disagree on what an animal's best interests are. For example, because pain is a perception that is much more easily examined in verbal animals, veterinarians disagree on how to evaluate and relieve an animal's pain.[6] Thus, even when clients and veterinarians hold similar views on the value of animals and the responsibility owed to pets, they may still disagree on what counts as health and illness or a good or bad quality of life.

As noted in Chapters 4 and 5, some ethical tensions and problems of the rookie are easily solved with time and experience, but others are not. In these chapters we see how veterinarians cope when unable to resolve tensions in their role. Ideally, veterinarians have an economically sustainable business, help sick animals by doing what they think is best for them, and have good relationships with clients and colleagues. However, many participants found themselves prioritizing one desire at the expense of another. Veterinarians had difficulty when their role in euthanasia caused moral conflict.[7] As discussed in Chapters 1 and 5, although veterinarians developed many problem-based and emotion-based coping strategies, even experienced veterinarians continued to feel tension in the interpretation of their professional role in life-and-death decision making.

The traditional role of the veterinarian has been to merely provide a list of options for clients that vary in cost, quality, and sophistication so that clients can decide what services they want. However, the role of the modern companion-animal veterinarian is changing because veterinarians are not always willing to leave decisions entirely up to the owner. Increasingly, they advocate for the best interests of animals just as pediatricians advocate for the best interests of children. When describing professional roles for veterinarians, Bernard Rollin juxtaposes what he calls a pediatrician model with a mechanic model.[8] In the mechanic model, the animal is likened to a car; the mechanic owes nothing to the car and fixes it or not depending on the owner's wishes. Each perspective leads to a different approach to guiding clients: paternalistically directing clients or respecting the client's autonomy to make decisions for their own animals.

Participants differed as to how much authority veterinarians should have over decisions made regarding pet animals. For some participants a veterinarian's job is to advocate for the patient, but ultimately the decision rests in the hands of a client, who is the customer. As one veterinarian said, "This animal belongs to someone else who has the right to decide the fate of their animal, and I may not agree with their choice, but I have to respect it." For other participants a veterinarian's job is to offer information to clients, who pay the bills. But they often take more of an advocacy role for the patient, as this veterinarian argued: "Medical situations often involve subjective interpretation, so I may downplay certain things or play up certain things in how I present information, because I am the expert. So clients are coming to me for my evaluation of what is best for their animal." Regardless of their stance on how much authority they believe a client should have in life-and-death decisions, nearly every veterinarian had a limit to the authority they were willing to give clients. For example, when it came to the question of the euthanasia of healthy animals, nearly every participant held firm against this request.

In general, some veterinarians placed a higher value on respecting the client's autonomy, while others felt justified in being more paternalistic and convincing clients to follow a certain course of action. Most participants landed somewhere along a continuum between the pediatrician and the mechanic models. They believed that veterinarians have a commitment to respect the choices of clients but should also be an advocate for patients. Most found their role changeable, complex, and multifaceted. For example, most participants placed a high value on client autonomy but found paternalism mandatory at times. Although many interns began their first year in practice closer to the pediatrician end of the continuum, by the end of their internships almost all of the interns were near the center.

Just as participants argued that they were neither completely a mechanic (allowing clients full autonomy) nor completely a pediatrician (insisting on a paternalistic approach), Clinton Sanders argues that companion animals fall along a continuum somewhere between objects and individuals, between persons and nonpersons.[9] He notes that a strict dichotomy between subject and object is false, as nonhuman animals are not simply objects to be dominated nor are they subjects with the same rights and moral status as humans. For veterinarians the animal is both patient and property, thus they serve the health of the patient and the client who pays the bill. However, as seen throughout the book, differences in the moral status of animals lead to conflicts and disagreements between veterinarians and their clients that are often difficult to resolve. Veterinarians worked diligently to balance their commitments to patients and clients, arguing with owners at times but also working to find a way to understand the owner's perspective.

Animals as Property: Elements of the Mechanic

As Rollin might have predicted, the vast majority of participants believed that adherence to the pediatrician model was the moral ideal for their profession. However, they also realized how far the profession was from being able to achieve that ideal. Because their patients are legally property and veterinarians depend on clients for income, participants recognized elements of the mechanic model inherent in their job. For example, when negotiating with owners over the cost and extent of medical treatment, veterinarians often literally compare their job to that of a mechanic or a used-car salesman:

> You are trained to offer them the Cadillac version of everything, and when that doesn't work, you come on down until you finally get to the 1969 Volkswagen version of treatment or even the Ford Pinto of treatment plans. When they say they can't afford it, I just give them the option B. You kind of negotiate it. . . . What [treatment] can I do without and still help this animal? Of course, you always want them to buy the Cadillac, but that is a really hard line to walk because they may end up just euthanizing if you don't offer them enough options.

At the same time, as the following veterinarian explained, participants also feel obligated to their clients:

> At least if I were a mechanic, I could give an estimate, and the car would run, and I could fulfill my end of the bargain. Sometimes people spend lots of money and the animal dies or we can't fix it. It is a lot of pressure on us. You are just left feeling like you wish you could have given them a happy ending since they have spent like $7,000.

However, as mentioned previously, putting themselves into the category of either pediatrician or mechanic seemed just as ill fitting as putting their patients into the category of either property or person:

> Plus, it is not simply being a mechanic in the strictest sense of the word. I bet my mechanic doesn't get emotionally attached to the cars

he works on. If it is an animal that I really want to treat for some reason [or] I am really attached to the owner or the pet, then I am a little
bit more, I guess, emotional about it.

Thus, participants believed the pediatrician model was the ethical ideal, but they
could not deny that parts of the mechanic model were inherent in their jobs.

Because animals are legally considered property and veterinarians depend
on clients for income, veterinary medicine is more client oriented than patient
oriented from both a legal and practical standpoint. Although unsavory at
times, bargaining and open negotiation of treatment expense is a reality in
veterinary medicine:

> Owners will sometimes say to me, "What can you do for a hundred
> bucks?" I feel like I am a used car dealer. I can offer you this nice
> Cadillac, or we have this nice Ford Pinto over here for a hundred
> dollars. . . . It becomes very much like the animal becomes forgotten
> and you are just, like, talking about money and negotiating treat-
> ment. Sometimes I think, "What the hell? We might as well offer our
> services on eBay."

As you can see from the tone of the quotation, veterinarians may identify
with the mechanic model but also find it frustrating. The veterinarian has
expert knowledge, but the client must be willing to pay for it. When clients
complain that they cannot pay for the veterinarian's suggestions, veterinarians must negotiate the types of services they will provide and perhaps even
haggle over their cost. Thus, the veterinarian's role can seem closer to an auto
mechanic's than a medical practitioner's.

In the United States both medical and veterinary professionals must
generate income when providing care for their patients, but in veterinary
medicine the bottom line rests on owners' ability and willingness to pay
for treatment rather than insurance companies or state-funded hospitals.[10]
Veterinary practices often have to enforce payment by requiring a deposit:
"The financial reality is different in veterinary medicine compared to human
stuff—not that I think dealing with managed care is any easier, but I really
can't do anything without money. I just can't do anything. You can't treat for
free." Another participant explained her frustration with what she sees as the
differences between medical and veterinary practices:

> What we can do for the pet is governed by the owner's willingness
> and owner finances. . . . Our patients deserve quality health care,

but euthanasia lurks over our head. . . . If you got in a car accident, . . . before they even knew if you had health insurance they would have an IV in you and you would be getting fluids. Whereas here a dog . . . hit by a car sits in the exam room, and you have to show them your credit card before you can get IV fluids. We are totally dependent on the owner. It is the nature of this field, and it can be very frustrating.

Although many novice interns found negotiating the financial aspects of veterinary medicine incompatible with their concept of medical provider to patients, scholars argue they must change their mind-set: "The attitude that any concern for monetary reward is not in true keeping with the professional spirit may be admirable, but it ignores the reality that financial success is a vital prerequisite to professional success."[11]

Veterinarians who believe their expertise is equal to that of physicians' are frustrated that they can charge only one-tenth of their counterparts' fees and often do not receive the respect they believe their profession deserves. Participants often compared their work to that of medical doctors with disappointment: "We do the same things as medical doctors but for a lot less money. We score higher on the MCATs [Medical College Admission Tests] and have to learn the same physiology but on a whole host of species. We have the same amount of education they do and the same debt, but we work for a lot less, and we get a lot less respect." Another veterinarian commented, "Sometimes people don't even know that we are *real* doctors. We worked just as hard as doctors for just as long, but people think, because our patients are animals, that we don't deserve the same respect."

Unlike principles of human medicine that assume all patients are in some sense equal in value, in veterinary medicine there is considerable disagreement about the value of patients.[12] Larry Carbone suggests, "To many people, veterinary medicine is much closer to agriculture and to dog shows than to human medicine. It is *animal* medicine, not animal *medicine*."[13] Veterinarians arguably have similar training and as large a body of expert knowledge as medical professionals, yet they earn significantly less income.[14] As recently as the 1970s, veterinary income was close to that of other medical professionals, including physicians; however, today the average annual income of physicians is nearly double the average annual salary of full-time veterinarians.[15] Moreover, while both veterinarians and medical professionals are hit with high tuition costs and student loan debt, veterinarians use a larger percentage of their monthly wages to pay off their debt (10 percent for veterinarians and 5 percent for physicians).[16]

The power dynamics of doctor-patient relationships have received considerable attention,[17] but veterinarian-client relationships remain relatively unexamined. For example, the physician is observed to have more power relative to the patient, who is typically rendered subservient to the physician's authority and instruction. However, Julius Roth suggests veterinarians lack the same kinds of freedoms medical doctors enjoy because "veterinarians do what their clients want even though they may consider it absurd, unnecessary, or even immoral because the veterinarian answers directly to the client (owner) rather than the patient (animal)."[18]

Because veterinarians are more likely to be subject to client demands, veterinarians are what Eliot Freidson calls client-dependent professionals.[19] The client-dependent practitioner is "quite isolated from his colleagues and relatively free of their control but at the same time he is very vulnerable to control by his clients. To keep them, he must give them what they want or someone else will."[20] To be chosen again, the client-dependent practice "must be prepared to provide services that honor the client's prejudices sufficiently to make him feel that what he thinks bothers him is being treated properly."[21] Participants all recognized that they were subject to client controls, as this participant summarized, "We have to remember that this is not an animal profession but a people profession that happens to be in the service of animals."

The conflicting professional and business elements of veterinarians' work—they serve both a patient and a customer—cause them frustration. When animals were euthanized because of financial limitations, owners blamed high veterinary bills and greedy veterinarians for their animal's fate: "They start to get really upset with you when you say that you have to have a deposit before we pursue treatment. They are like, 'What are you, heartless? Don't you care that my dog needs this?'" The cover story of the June 2004 issue of *Veterinary Economics* addressed the issue of veterinarians who feel pulled between the desire to care for patients and the need to make money for their practice: "When we say we can't afford to keep giving away free or reduced services and products, we're met with mistrust that sometimes borders on loathing. . . . [W]e are private practitioners and business owners?"[22] Participants also complained of suspicions from some clients regarding financing their animal's care: "The nerve of these people questioning me with such distrust, asking in a huff, 'Well, how much is that going to cost me?' I am a fucking doctor for fuck's sake, and I drive a freaking base-model Kia. I don't deserve this kind of attitude."

Some participants argued that perhaps the veterinary profession has not been effective in conveying to the public the monetary value of the service that is involved in treating animals. One hospital administrator described encouraging interns to see their work as valuable and the cost of service justifiable:

> We try to explain to the interns that we are not just nagging them about their records and charges because we need to recoup our financial costs. We are nagging them about charging owners for what they do because their work is valuable and people should pay for the service we provide. It is really hard for the interns to learn this.

Although many novices started out fairly timid when addressing the cost of treatments, they grew more and more confident and even learned to justify the cost of treatment to owners:

> It does get easier to look an owner in the eye and tell them it is going to be five grand. It is tough at first, but it gets easier. You have to start to have some real backbone, but also you have to be secure in yourself knowing that the services that you are offering are worth it. You have to know that this is a sick patient and they are going to need a lot of care, and I see how much care all of the staff and all of the doctors are going to put into this animal, and we deserve to get paid for our services, and this is me doing a lot of work, and it is worth this amount.

Yet even participants with years of experience had difficulty reconciling their healing and pecuniary roles. In fact, some hesitated to offer the best for their patients because the client might question their motivations in diagnostic and treatment recommendations.

The stress associated with financial issues in veterinary care highlights the difficulties that many participants had in trying to step outside the mechanic model. The pediatrician model requires the veterinary profession to convey to the public that animals are worthy of expensive medical treatment. Veterinary ethicists such as Bernard Rollin encourage veterinarians to use their medical authority for the benefit of the animal.[23] David Main argues that veterinarians need not be hesitant or embarrassed in advocating for expensive treatment if it is in the best interest of the animal.[24] In their discussions of ethical issues associated with the provision of veterinary services, practitioners and ethicists alike stress the need for dialogue with respect to veterinarians' responsibilities to both animals and clients.[25] They raise questions for the profession to help clinicians reflect on their actions and resolve ethical tension in positive, ethically consistent ways that benefit clients, patients, and themselves.

Animals as Patients: Elements of the Pediatrician

Because their patients are legally considered property, participants found themselves limited in their ability to follow a pediatrician model. However, that the law treats nonhuman animals strictly as property is increasingly problematic for many Americans.[26] Because of the legal status of animals, it is difficult to prosecute acts of malfeasance toward them, and punitive damages are limited to a nebulously defined market value.[27] For example, law professor Anna Charlton describes an incident in Michigan in which a woman's mixed-breed dog was severely injured by a delivery truck.[28] When the apologetic business owner submitted the $400 in veterinary bills to his insurance company, it refused to pay the full amount. The company argued against payment on the grounds that the dog was not worth the money and should have been considered "totaled," as in the case of a severely damaged automobile. If the estimated cost to fix a car is more than its value, it is considered totaled and the insurance company pays the owner its value rather than the expense of the repairs. For many people cases such as these demonstrate flaws in the legal status of animals. They argue that pet animals are fundamentally different from inanimate property and call for the creation of a special category of property that differentiates animals as living property.[29]

The perception of the importance of companion animals is changing and veterinarians are taking notice. An article in the journal *Veterinary Economics* examines the changing status of pets, noting that courts increasingly recognize animals as greater than simply property and that their lives should be counted as more valuable than their market value.[30] Some people are lobbying for pet owners to be defined as *guardians* rather than *owners* of their animal companions.[31] Because it is difficult to predict how these changes in societal attitudes and legislation will influence the veterinary profession, speculation abounds.[32] For example, the more pets are treated as surrogate children, the more some veterinarians fear an increase in malpractice suits; others are excited by the possible economic benefits for veterinarians. Indeed, research conducted by the American Veterinary Medical Association suggests that the intensity of the human-animal bond may play a central role in a pet owner's decision to seek veterinary care. In its 2006 survey, nearly half of pet owners considered their pets to be family members.[33] Households that consider their dogs and cats to be family members averaged more than 3 veterinary visits per year, households with pets or companions averaged 2.2 visits, and those that consider pets to be property averaged only 1 visit. In other words, this evidence suggests that the animal's status within the family has a close association with number of veterinary visits and total spending on veterinary care.

Veterinary medicine is indeed a profession undergoing many significant changes. Today, the great majority of veterinary students are females[34] who will treat companion animals.[35] A generation ago, veterinarians were overwhelmingly males who focused on the treatment of economically valuable farm animals;[36] women were thought to lack the necessary strength or stamina for the job.[37] In the 1960s women were just 5 percent of veterinary students, and it wasn't until the 1970s and 1980s that they began entering veterinary medicine in significant numbers.[38] Since 1983 female applicants to U.S. veterinary schools have outnumbered male applicants.[39] Today, half of all practicing veterinarians in the United States are women, and nearly 80 percent of students at the twenty-eight veterinary schools in the United States are women.[40] The proportion of female graduates of veterinary colleges is so large it exceeds that of other professional groups such as physicians, lawyers, and engineers, professions in which men continue to outnumber women in both degree programs and as practicing professionals.[41]

The level of care that is possible for small-animal veterinarians to provide to their patients is also rapidly evolving and expanding. In a study of euthanasia with death and dying as its focus, it is possible to lose sight of the big picture for my study's participants. Although this book does not give much consideration to the rewards of veterinary medicine as a whole, I can attest to the personal joy of helping sick animals recover and solving difficult diagnostic challenges, as well as the thrill of watching unique surgeries and the use of amazing technologies. Because of technological advances and the willingness of some pet owners to invest financially in their pet's health and well-being, today's veterinarians offer treatments older generations only dreamed of providing their patients. Companion-animal veterinarians have exciting jobs in which they can specialize in over thirty subfields, including cardiology, radiology, ophthalmology, and oncology. Increasingly, animals receive advanced medical, dental, and surgical care, including dialysis, root canals, hip replacements, chemotherapy, cataract extractions, and even pacemakers. In the words of one participant, as he used a video endoscopic tool to search for and grab an object swallowed by one of his patients, "Today's veterinarians get to do some really cool shit."

Evidence from my research suggests veterinarians are thinking differently about their patients' subjective feelings. A key part of the typical negotiation process for the veterinarian is helping owners evaluate an animal's quality of life. Traditionally, determining when an animal's life has deteriorated enough to warrant euthanasia is based on observable signs of health and illness (e.g., eating, drinking, urinating and defecating, and breathing difficulty) and objective medical procedures (e.g., blood tests, radiographs, and ultrasound). Of course, all veterinarians continue to use this objective approach; however, a growing number also include subjective measures in an attempt to evaluate a pet's happiness or general satisfaction with life (e.g., would Buster be happy if he could no longer do his favorite activities, and does he have the psychological makeup to withstand painful treatments?).

This new subjective approach to evaluating quality of life for animals is often problematic because no universally agreed on standards exist for determining the subjective feelings of other animals and veterinary experts can reach vastly different conclusions when judging an animal's objective or subjective quality of life. This book does not debate how or what animals think and feel. However, what is most interesting to me is that both veterinarians and their clients are beginning to include mental issues in determining an animal's quality of life.[42] By assuming that nonhuman animals have the capacity for a subjective experience, veterinarians and pet owners are placing companion animals in a category closer to personhood.

Many veterinarians are calling for their leading veterinary organization, the American Veterinary Medical Association (AVMA), to become a stronger advocate for animals. For example, some veterinarians want animal welfare to be incorporated in the veterinary curriculum,[43] while others argue that veterinarians should take leadership roles in shaping animal welfare policies and addressing animal cruelty.[44] Many of these practitioners would like to see the AVMA's *Principles of Veterinary Medical Ethics* do more to ensure animal welfare.[45] While most participants supported the organization's stance on the responsible use of animals for companionship, work, production, food, teaching, research, and recreation and sport, as well as wild animal management, their definition of *responsible* received much debate. For example, debate is ongoing within the profession over whether declawing cats, debarking dogs, housing sows in gestation crates, and keeping egg-laying poultry hens in factory farms constitute responsible treatment of animals.

Participants often reported disagreement with the AVMA regarding approved practices, including ear cropping and tail docking, declawing of cats, use of terminal surgeries (described later) in veterinary school, and euthanasia of healthy animals without regard to medical necessity. While some participants raised purebred animals, they often opposed breed standards for certain animals when the standards require cosmetic surgical intervention to dock long tails or clip floppy ears (e.g., for Doberman pinschers). The practice of onychectomy,[46] or cat declawing, was morally problematic for several participants, who felt it results in pain and distress without medical benefit to the animal. A few participants provided these surgeries without comment, others only under specific circumstances, but most outright refused.

Several participants expressed concerns that the veterinary ethical code has no explicit requirement mandating that euthanasia be in the recipient's best interest or serve primarily to alleviate suffering. The principles of veterinary ethics make only one statement regarding euthanasia, that "humane euthanasia of animals is an ethical veterinary procedure."[47] One particularly controversial practice is the so-called convenience euthanasia, so named because it is for owner convenience rather than for medical or behavioral reasons.[48] The term alone is controversial because it is difficult to define and because some consider it a slur against fellow veterinarians who choose to euthanize healthy animals. However, in response to the controversy, many veterinary practices have implemented policies regarding what should be done when an owner seeks euthanasia for reasons the veterinarian does not support.

One of the most controversial parts of veterinary education is terminal surgeries, known to medical and veterinary students as dog lab. Although conduct of these laboratory classes can vary widely, they usually involve assigning an animal to a group of two or three students who perform specific surgeries on the animal over several weeks and then euthanize the animal.[49] Young veterinarians increasingly voice disagreement with this controversial educational technique.[50] Some veterinary schools defend the practice as teaching valuable skills that will later be used to help save many animals' lives, but others have banned the class or made it optional to conscientious objectors. Educators are increasingly developing and relying on alternatives to the use of animals, such as computer models and simulations.[51] Although the use of live animals in veterinary school is a controversial issue beyond this scope of this book, controversies such as these are manifestations of the growing conflict between traditional ethics and newly emerging attitudes and values. Students entering veterinary schools most often mention the "desire to work with and care for animals" when asked to define the most important reason they want to become a veterinarian.[52] Given that these students accord greater importance to animal welfare than did veterinarians in earlier times, researchers predict they will continue to bring these issues to the forefront of veterinary medicine.[53]

Chapters 2 and 3 reveal a growing commitment among veterinarians to recognize the intense feelings of grief, pain, and sorrow resulting from the death of a pet. These veterinarians do their best to make the euthanasia process as painless as possible for the animal and as peaceful as possible for the grieving pet owner. Although emotion work was not as easy for some participants as others, even they clearly got involved in their clients' emotions. Clients who would normally be considered problematic time sinks or high-maintenance "animal nuts"[54] were often indulged during euthanasia procedures. Some participants even went to clients' homes or to a favorite park for euthanasia, and although exceptional, a rare few attended funeral ceremonies or gatherings after the euthanasia:

> I have done at-home euthanasia. One of them I was there for two hours. . . . The woman was really great, and that cat—I just loved that cat. And it was just so sad. . . . And we were sitting in the garden. It was nice. . . . He was just walking around sniffing the grass, and then he'd lie down in the grass and look around. And she had one of these beautiful gardens where there were birds everywhere. So he was watching the birds. . . . It was really special. . . . And obviously, I don't have that time with all clients, but there are those clients or there are those situations where you do that kind of thing.

Although some veterinarians consider such emotion work outside the domain of knowledge, experience, and responsibility of veterinarians, participants patiently and tirelessly helped clients deal with the emotional watershed that often accompanies the death of a pet.

The details of Chapters 2 and 3 also underscore the importance of human-animal bonds for many of today's pet owners. We see companion animals as much closer to subjects than objects—more like members of the family. When confronted with end-of-life decisions for beloved companion animals, pet owners can feel intense grief over the loss of strong bonds with their animals. Participants were often surprised at the intensity of people's emotions: "They say some pretty private things. You really get to see how much people love their animals. It is just their raw emotion and they say things. It can get really intense." As much as the practice of euthanasia can be physically and emotionally demanding, frustrating, and disappointing, it can be extraordinarily rewarding for the veterinarian. Through this experience, veterinarians get a bird's-eye view of the special emotional relationships that people share with nonhuman animals.

Many participants strongly argued that dealing with client emotions is essential to providing client satisfaction and building long-term relationships with them. In response to the increasingly strong bonds clients share with their animals and to changes in client demand regarding the death of their animals, the profession is concerning itself more with human-animal bonds. Veterinarians are beginning to develop bond-centered practices that focus not just on the medical care of animals but also on the emotional well-being of the client.[55] These veterinarians are calling for courses devoted to grief management and to the study of the human-animal bond to become a standard part of the veterinary curriculum.[56] In addition, by memorializing and ritualizing companion animals' deaths, veterinarians reinforce the notion that animals are worthy of such honor, ceremony, and human grief. Of course, by extension, such acts of veneration are also a sign that companion animals are worth the cost of expensive medical care. Veterinarians increasingly advocate for quality health care as a responsibility of every pet owner. Several bumper stickers I saw on vehicles in a staff parking lot comically recognized this fact: "The other family doctor—your veterinarian."

Appendix

Methodology

This discussion draws on data gathered through approximately eighteen months of ethnographic research in two large veterinary teaching hospitals renowned for excellence in training veterinary professionals in the northeastern region of the United States. Because of the enthusiasm of key veterinary insiders regarding my research interests, I had access to multiple veterinary hospitals. My initial fieldwork consisted of three months in a veterinary teaching hospital in New York State. From that experience, I was invited to attend several classes at a New England veterinary college, including a half-day seminar on euthanasia. Next, my fieldwork at a teaching hospital in Massachusetts coincided with their thirteen-month internship program. Last, I compared what I had learned in the Northeast with fieldwork in an emergency veterinary hospital in Santa Barbara, California.

Immersed in the day-to-day activities of doctors of veterinary medicine (DVMs), I observed their interactions with human clients, animal patients, technicians, and colleagues. Throughout my graduate school training I was fortunate to be able to go back and forth between analyzing the data I had earlier collected and spending time in the field among veterinarians. This allowed me to use the inductive process of grounded theory in my analysis.[1] In essence, grounded theory attempts to reach a theory or conceptual understanding through inductive processes. Research questions begin the inquiry, and the researcher constantly compares themes that emerge from the data with earlier expectations and assumptions. After each set of interviews,

I modified the interview guide and developed questions for follow-up interviews based on recursive analysis of the themes that emerged from the initial interviews and field observations.[2] In this way, the researcher's own theories and insights are firmly grounded in participants' narratives and observable experiences.

One important criticism of ethnographic methods is that, because samples tend to be small and not chosen by randomized sampling techniques, the conclusions drawn from fieldwork cannot be generalized. Given that my study's participants were not selected in a way to represent all veterinarians, I do not claim to offer an objective, broadly generalizable view of veterinary euthanasia as it is practiced everywhere in the United States. I limited my study to small-animal, or companion-animal, veterinarians focusing on the treatment of pet dogs, cats, gerbils, birds, reptiles, rabbits, and other animals; however, between 65 and 70 percent of U.S. veterinarians' earnings in 2008 came from treating small animals.[3] While some veterinarians work in mixed-animal practices where they might see pigs, goats, horses, and sheep in addition to companion animals, less than 15 percent of veterinarians work exclusively in large-animal practices.

Perhaps what sets the majority of my study's participants apart from the typical veterinarian is that they practice in large, urban teaching hospitals. While the vast majority of American veterinarians practice in small, locally owned clinics immediately upon graduation from veterinary school, teaching hospitals host elective, advanced training programs that require many hours and intense dedication from students. With state-of-the-art technology and board-certified specialists, they usually offer clients the most sophisticated veterinary care available in their area, including emergency or critical care; ophthalmology, neurology, and oncology services; and cardiovascular and orthopedic surgery. In addition to these sophisticated services, however, teaching hospitals also provide the same preventive and basic health care offered by most small-animal clinicians. Thus teaching hospitals exposed me to a large number of clients seeking care for animal patients with a wide variety of medical conditions.

Though teaching hospitals are somewhat atypical veterinary clinics, they advantageously exposed me to a large number of veterinarians. I captured a wide range of perspectives, from those of novices fresh out of veterinary school to those of skilled specialists with nearly forty years of experience, ranging in age from twenty-five to sixty-two. Although participants were 70 percent female, the demographics of my settings reflect the significant gender changes in the profession.[4] Women make up approximately half of practicing veterinarians and nearly 80 percent of veterinary students. Given that teaching hospitals host a large number of residents and interns who recently graduated from veterinary school, I expected to have a greater percentage of female participants. All told, my data consist of eighty-one formal interviews with fifty-four veterinarians and over six hundred hours of observation.

Participants included veterinarians from many of the twenty-eight schools of veterinary medicine in the United States, including Cornell, Ohio State University, Purdue, Texas A&M, Tufts University, University of California at Davis, University of Georgia, University of Illinois at Urbana-Champaign, University of Pennsylvania, and Washington State University. I also attended several veterinary conferences where I spoke with practitioners from all over the country whose perspectives closely reflected those of my study's participants. Although the demographics of this group do not represent all veterinarians, I believe that the experiences presented in the book will resonate for veterinarians around the country. Indeed, my time in a California clinic confirmed that many thoughts, feelings, and experiences I learned of on the East Coast were similar to those of the West. That my findings were consistent across multiple settings suggests they are credible beyond the specific organizational culture of one hospital.

Another methodological concern of ethnographic investigators has to do with the influence of the researcher on the behavior of those observed. In other words, researchers may influence the accuracy of their findings or participants may alter their behavior while observed, working to present themselves in the most favorable light.[5] During my research there were many indications that my presence did not significantly alter the actions of the participants.

First, I believe my presence was minimally invasive as my fieldwork did not interfere in the daily operations of the hospitals. Taking advantage of the teaching hospital setting, I essentially played the role of a pseudostudent shadowing clinical staff. My fieldwork was not especially conspicuous to veterinary participants or their clients because veterinary students often take notes and record data in these settings. Moreover, staff members employed in teaching hospitals are relatively accustomed to having students in their workspace for extended periods who express diligent interest in their work. Some participants became so accustomed to my presence that, more than once, I had to remind them I was not actually a veterinary insider and could not possibly answer the technical questions they directed my way.

The character of my research interests meant that I could not avoid interactions with emotionally vulnerable clients. Although staff members knew me as a researcher, clients were never told of this identity and most likely were never aware of their role in my research. When interacting with clients, I was introduced by most veterinarians simply by name or generically as a student observer; others did not refer to me at all. Clients most likely assumed I was a veterinary technician because I often borrowed laboratory coats, dressed in hospital scrubs, and helped veterinarians with simple tasks. Although this aspect of my fieldwork was often uncomfortable and sometimes emotionally upsetting, I took care to observe unobtrusively, with sensitivity and respect appropriate to the situation.

Second, I am confident I obtained reliable information because I was with the participants for a long time. During my time at the hospitals, I observed as many cases as possible on day, evening, and overnight shifts. I attended clinical rotations in emergency and critical care and oncology and occasionally sat in on internal medicine, ophthalmology, gastroenterology, respiratory medicine, neurology, cardiology, dermatology, and avian-exotic medicine rounds. Throughout my research I saw both unusual and common cases, including broken bones, collapsed tracheas, heartworm, ingested foreign bodies, motor dysfunction, anorexia, various toxicities, urinary blockages, and lots and lots of vomiting and diarrhea. I spent many long days with frustrated veterinarians whose canine patients, especially Labradors, swallowed just about anything they could get their paws on. But at the same time, I was alongside participants when they solved difficult cases and made heroic saves. In other words, my presence was fairly ubiquitous. Sharing ordinary as well as extraordinary experiences with participants helped establish my genuine interest in their work.

Finally, extensive documentation shows that having rapport with participants facilitates authentic data collection.[6] I built rapport with participants by spending long hours them and by sharing in the daily grind of the profession. My typical involvement included cleaning examination tables, bathing animals, transporting patients and delivering their charts around the hospital, and monitoring equipment. On occasion, I assisted in noncritical procedures such as restraining patients or taking their temperatures. In one memorable incident I sustained a semiserious injury while helping restrain a very agitated domestic short-haired cat. After the feline patient rudely dug her back claws into my arm, staff members cleaned my wounds and commiserated with me regarding such work-related hazards. Admittedly, I proudly displayed my injuries by wearing short sleeves all week in hopes that others would notice my wounds and interpret the injury as a sign of my commitment to the project.

As time when on, it became clear to me that getting my hands dirty with participants helped them feel at ease with me. I became especially adept at an unpopular task known as expressing anal glands. Without going into detail, suffice it to say that the oily secretions gently coaxed out of the swollen gland have a very disagreeable odor to humans. Thankfully, the sometimes painful and pungent tasks helped build rapport with participants, which facilitated discussion of emotionally uncomfortable work-related experiences.

Humor also aided my transition from outsider status to acceptance in the private workspace of veterinarians. As I describe in Chapter 5, participants publicly analyzed my character through the telling and retelling of two particularly embarrassing events that happened to me early in my fieldwork. My willingness to laugh at these emotionally troubling and embarrassing situations reinforced my reputation as someone who can withstand the difficult parts of the job and who can be trusted with sensitive, insider information. Similar to Teela Sanders's experience as a researcher among sex workers, in every setting I became the source of jokes, gags, and funny stories aimed at testing my willingness to play along.[7] For example, because of my research interest in euthanasia, participants often playfully implied that I was macabre or enjoyed being present for euthanasia procedures. They teased me by saying, "Oh, you missed a sad one today," or "You should have been following me last night 'cause I killed everything that walked in the door!" The interns especially enjoyed making me the butt of the joke by asking me technical questions in front of clients so that they could later take mischievous pleasure in my awkward and unscientific responses. Although such teasing may seem harsh and alienating to some readers, it made me feel welcome. Moreover, workplace researchers repeatedly note humor as a key part of socializing newcomers, relieving tension, and building a sense of group camaraderie.[8] Participating in playful repartee and good-humored teasing not only reinforced my acceptance as an insider; it also helped participants become more comfortable with me (and helped me become more comfortable with them).

Throughout the research process, I cultivated a collegial relationship with all participants, and I believe that most came to see me as a person they could trust and who understood their dilemmas. No other time was this more apparent than when participants broke hospital policy in my presence. Although most infractions were relatively minor, such as processing blood or urine samples without charging clients, such behavior could result in censure if reported to hospital administrators. A few violations I witnessed were far more serious. For example, veterinarians could lose their license for contracting with a client to euthanize a pet and not following through with that agreement. On more than one occasion, I watched as participants saved animals from euthanasia by giving them to other people without the previous owner's knowledge or consent. To ease fear of exposure I often reminded them that I would hold our conversations and interactions in strict confidence and I would not use their real names or give details that could lead to their identification.

Eventually, participants came to see me as a person they could confide in, and I became more and more certain that I could trust what I saw and heard as genuine. Some participants shared more freely than others, and as time went on several clearly saw me as a person to talk to about their work and eagerly included me in anything related to euthanasia. Participants increasingly brought up sensitive matters without my prodding and sometimes went out of their way to find me in the hospital to share events they thought relevant to the project. For example, after noticing my interest in the euthanasia-related cards, letters, and gifts displayed around their offices, participants often saved them to show me during our interviews.

While no employees refused to allow me to observe them at work, I was unable to schedule formal interviews with every veterinarian employed at the hospitals because of time constraints. Given my participants' demanding schedules, a few of the interviews took place in break rooms or hallways during slow shifts. In most cases, however, the interviews took place while participants were off duty in isolated areas of the hospital such as the library or a private office. Most interviews lasted approximately one hour, but some lasted for as long as three hours. Although my fieldwork was often emotionally upsetting and physically exhausting, ethnographic methods gave me direct access to the private and emotionally charged interactions between veterinarians and their clients not possible through standardized questionnaires.

Notes

INTRODUCTION

1. Proponents of ethnographic methods argue that researchers learn the most about a group (or culture) when they are able to observe and participate in group activity and conduct interviews with group members (Tope et al. 2005; Taylor and Bogdan 1998; VanMaanen 1988). Only through long-term immersion in a group can researchers solidly ground their theories and analysis in the group's stories and observable experiences (Berg 2004; Lofland et al. 2005). See the Appendix for a description of my research method.

2. Kilarski 2003.

3. For example, see Arluke and Sanders 1996; Burghardt and Herzog 1989; Franklin 1999; Hal Herzog 2010; Irvine 2004; Manning and Serpell 1994.

4. Lawrence 1988.

5. Serpell 2009.

6. Wilkie 2010.

7. C. Sanders 1999.

8. Arluke 1991b, 1994a; Phillips 1993, 1994; Wolfle 1985.

9. Arluke and Sanders 1996.

10. Arluke 1991a; Irvine 2004.

11. Case 1991.

12. Arluke 2004b; Arluke and Hafferty 1996.

13. Arluke 2004a.

14. Hal Herzog 2010.

15. As found in Harold Herzog 1993.

16. Arluke and Sanders 1996.

17. Swabe 2000.

18. Doherty and Feeney 2004.

19. Albert and Bulcroft 1988; Cain 1983; Gosse and Barnes 1994; Katcher 1989; Voith 1985.

20. Cohen 2002a.

21. American Veterinary Medical Association 2007.

22. Bilger 2003.

23. Atwood-Harvey 2005.

24. Arluke and Sanders 1996.

25. Emanuel 1994; Gaylin et al. 1988; Nyman, Eidelman, and Sprung 1996.

26. Cohen et al. 1994; Gianelli 1994; Greenberg 1997; Lee et al. 1996; Seale 2009.

27. Dr. Jack Kevorkian was the controversial advocate for a terminal patient's right to die via physician-assisted suicide; he assisted patients to that end and served eight years in prison for second-degree murder. Kevorkian (1991) discusses medicide in his book *Prescription Medicide: The Goodness of Planned Death*.

28. Seale 2009.

29. For example, see Rollin 1999; and Tannenbaum 1995.

30. Morgan and McDonald 2007.

31. Stanford and Keto 1991.

32. The two leading brands for animal euthanasia solution are Euthasol (manufactured by Virbac) and Fatal-Plus (manufactured by Vortech). Both solutions contain pentobarbital sodium as the active ingredient, but they use different dyes; Euthasol is pink, while Fatal-Plus is blue.

33. Rowe and Regehr 2010.

34. Pogrebin and Poole 1988; Scott 2007.

35. Tracy, Myers, and Scott 2006.

36. Astedt-Kurki and Liukkonen 1994; Harries 1995; Meerabeau and Page 1998; Wanzer, Booth-Butterfield, and Booth-Butterfield 2005.

37. Coombs et al. 1993; Gordon 1983; Hafferty 1991; Nelson 1992; Schulman-Green 2003; Smith and Kleinman 1989; Wear et al. 2006.

38. Coombs et al. 1993; Francis 1994; Francis, Monahan, and Berger 1999; Mallett 1993; Rowe and Regehr 2010; Scott 2007.

39. Coombs et al. 1993; Gordon 1983.

40. Arluke 1988.

41. Francis, Monahan, and Berger 1999; Mizrahi 1984; Rowe and Regehr 2010; Sayre 2001; Watson 2011; Wear et al. 2006.

42. Albert and Bulcroft 1988; Cain 1983; Gosse and Barnes 1994; Katcher 1989; Voith 1985.

43. De Lorenzo and Augustine 2004; Heath et al. 2001; Lowe et al. 2009; Nelson, Kurtz, and Hacker 1988.

44. Barker and Barker 1988; Beck and Katcher 1996; Carmack 1985.

45. Albert and Bulcroft 1988; Belk 1996; Cain 1983; Greenebaum 2004; Kurdek 2008, 2009.

46. Although a person's experience of grief following the death of a pet depends on his or her level of emotional attachment, pet death has become an increasingly significant stressor in the lives of pet owners (Adams, Bonnett, and Meek 2000; Brown, Richards, and Wilson 1996; Chur-Hansen 2010; Field et al. 2009; Fogle and Abrahamson 1990; Gosse and Barnes 1994, Planchon and Templer 1996; Podrazik et al. 2000; Stephens and Hill 1996; Stern 1996).

47. For example, see Arluke 1980; Becker et al. 1961; Bosk 1979; Fox 1989; Friedman and McDaniel 1998; Granfield and Koenig 2003; Merton, Reader, and Kendall 1957; Mizrahi 1986.

48. Arluke 1997.

49. For example, see Anspach 1993; Cahill 1999; Charmaz 1980; Glaser and Strauss 1965; Hafferty 1991; Henry 2004; Kearl 1989; Seymour 2001; Smith and Kleinman 1989; and Timmermans 2002.

50. For example, see Cameron 1990; Foster 1985; Gage and Gage 1994; Haddock and Matthews 1985; Lose 1979; Sharp 2005; Witiak 2004; and Younker and Fried 1976.

51. Croke 1999; Sawicki 1996.

52. Herriot 1972.

53. For exceptions, see Arluke 2004b; Atwood-Harvey 2004, 2005; Bryant 1979; Bryant and Snizek 1976; Carbone 2004; Gauthier 2001; Herzog, Vore, and New 1989; Irvine and Vermilya 2010; Roberts 2004; Roth 1994; C. Sanders 1994a, 1994b, 1999; Stanford and Keto 1991; and Swabe 1999.

54. Roth 1994; C. Sanders 1995, 1999; Swabe 2000.

CHAPTER 1

1. Newfield et al. 2000.
2. Self et al. 1991; Self, Safford, and Shelton 1988.
3. C. Sanders 1995.
4. A radiograph is another term for an X-ray image.
5. Stivers 1998.
6. C. Sanders 1995, 204.
7. Wojciechowska and Hewson 2005.
8. Antelyes 1991; Schoen 1991.
9. Coe, Adams, and Bonnett 2007; Klingborg and Klingborg 2007.
10. Wojciechowska and Hewson 2005.
11. Nogueira Borden et al. 2010; Shaw et al. 2008.
12. Shaw et al. 2008.
13. Bateman 2007.
14. Shaw and Lagoni 2007.
15. Shaw, Adams, and Bonnett 2004.
16. Milani 2004, 2006b, 2006c.
17. Chun and Garrett 2007.
18. Abood 2008; Cornell and Kopcha 2007.
19. Kurtz 2006; Martin 2006; Nogueira Borden et al. 2010.
20. Similar behavior was also found in Gauthier's (2001) study of occupational deviance in veterinary practice.
21. Because the majority of my study participants were not in private practice, I suspected that I would see more deviance motivated by economic rationale in a private practice, as noted by Gauthier (2001). Most of my study's participants were salaried rather than production based, as Gauthier's were, and I thus found different acts of deviance and unique justifications. For example, participants violated hospital rules by doing services for free, arguing that the hospital made enough money and would not suffer if they did not charge for some services.

22. Antelyes 1991.
23. Mallery et al. 1999.
24. Yeates and Main 2010.

CHAPTER 2

1. Howarth 1996.
2. Ibid.; Turner and Edgley 1976.
3. Arterial thromboembolism (ATE), the formation of a thrombus, or blood clot, within an artery, is a complication of heart disease that often strikes without warning. Like most cats with this condition, this cat was in obvious and considerable pain, as evidenced by excited behavior, frenzy, vocalization, rolling, and panting.
4. Agonal respiration is a sign of extreme medical distress and marked by gasping, labored breathing, and random vocalizations. Agonal respiration is almost always associated with great pain and sometimes referred to as the agony of death, or last breaths before death.
5. Goffman 1959.
6. Howarth 1996; Hyland and Morse 1995; Turner and Edgley 1976.
7. Manning 1982.
8. Pasko 2002.
9. Guerrier and Adib 2003.
10. Haas and Shaffir 1977.
11. Ulsperger and Paul 2002.
12. Friedman 1994.
13. Hochschild 1983.
14. Korczynski 2003.
15. Goffman 1959.
16. Ibid.
17. Ibid.
18. Hochschild 1983.
19. See Godwin 2004; Guerrier and Adib 2003; Korczynski 2003; Larson and Yao 2005; Lewis 2005; Manning 1982; and Pasko 2002.
20. Crawley 2004.
21. Lewis 2005; Stenross and Kleinman 1989; Sutton 1991.
22. Stenross and Kleinman 1989.
23. Goffman 1959.
24. Hochschild 1983.
25. Young 1990.
26. Brissett and Edgley 1990.
27. Ulsperger and Paul 2002.
28. Boles, Davis, and Tatro 1983.

CHAPTER 3

1. Bryant and Snizek 1976; S. Jones 2003.
2. Grier 2006.

3. Ibid.

4. As an example of one such article, see Bustad, Hines, and Leathers 1981.

5. Adams, Bonnett, and Meek 2000; Martin et al. 2004.

6. Hochschild 1979, 1983.

7. DeCoster 1997.

8. Groves 1978.

9. Coates and Lo 1990.

10. Fuller and Geis 1985.

11. For example, see Cahill and Eggleston 1994; DeCoster 1997; Francis 1994; Francis, Monahan, and Berger 1999; Holyfield and Fine 1997; L. Jones 1997; Rafaeli and Sutton 1991; Roberts and Smith 2002; and Thoits 1996.

12. Lois 2001.

13. Sutton 1991.

14. Lois 2001.

15. Francis 1994.

16. Swabe (1994) discusses the display of emotions in euthanasia encounters and how they differ from the everyday veterinary interaction between client and professional.

17. Lofland 1985.

18. Brabant 1997.

19. Adams, Bonnett, and Meek 2000; Brown, Richards, and Wilson 1996; Chur-Hansen 2010; Field et al. 2009; Fogle and Abrahamson 1990; Gosse and Barnes 1994, Planchon and Templer 1996; Stern 1996; Weirich 1988.

20. Gerwolls and Labott 1994; Hart, Hart, and Mader 1990.

21. Gage and Holcomb 1991.

22. Carmack 1985; Quackenbush 1985.

23. Wrobel and Dye 2003.

24. Hetts and Lagoni 1990; Stewart et al. 1985; Weisman 1991.

25. Hetts and Lagoni 1990; Meyers 2002; Ross and Baron-Sorenson 1998.

26. Hart, Hart, and Mader 1990.

27. Adams, Bonnett, and Meek 2000.

28. Meyers 2002.

29. Lois 2001.

30. Goffman 1963, 207.

31. Lois 2001, 155.

32. Ibid., 139.

33. Ibid., 152.

34. DeCoster 1997.

35. DeCoster 1997; Leif and Fox 1963.

36. Goffman 1959, 1967; Swabe 1994.

37. Goffman 1959.

38. Although Swabe (1994) highlights that the interactional breakdown is restored by display of emotions in euthanasia encounters, she does not explore how it is restored.

39. Goffman 1959, 1963.

40. Goffman 1963.

41. Goffman 1959.

42. Gregory and Keto 1991.
43. Pilgram 2010.
44. Hochschild 1983.
45. Goffman 1959.
46. Crawley 2004; Goodrum and Stafford 2003.
47. Cohen 1985; Dunn, Mehler, and Greenberg 2005; Hart and Hart 1987; Mercer 2007.
48. Lois 2001.
49. Ibid., 173.
50. Clark 1997.
51. Arluke and Sanders 1996.
52. Clark 1997, 131.
53. Barker and Barker 1988; Carmack 1985.
54. Chur-Hansen 2010; Hart, Hart, and Mader 1990; Morley and Fook 2005; Weisman 1991.
55. Doka 2002.
56. Meyers 2002.
57. Adams, Bonnett, and Meek 2000.
58. For example, see Arluke and Sanders 1996; Lawrence 1988; Serpell 2009; Swabe 2000.
59. Hochschild 1989.
60. Meyers 2002; Stephens and Hill 1996.
61. Pilgram 2010.

CHAPTER 4

1. Cohen-Salter et al. 2004; Gelberg and Gelberg 2005; Herzog, Vore, and New 1989.
2. Haas and Shaffir 1977, 1982.
3. Heath 2002.
4. Fogle and Abrahamson 1990; Gardner and Hini 2006; Rollin 1987; C. Sanders 1995; Strand, Zaparanick, and Brace 2005.
5. C. Sanders 1995.
6. Heath 1997; Strand, Zaparanick, and Brace 2005.
7. Clark and LaBeff 1982; Ptacek, Leonard, and McKee 2004.
8. Chun and Garrett 2007; Wensley 2008.
9. Williams, and Mills 2000; Williams, Arnold, and Mills 2005.
10. Chiappetta-Swanson 2005; Field 1998; Redinbaugh et al. 2003; Wippen and Canellos 1991.
11. Heath and Lanyon 1996; Heath, Lynch-Blosse, and Lanyon 1996a.
12. Tannenbaum 1995.
13. Doka 2002; Meyers 2002.
14. Field 1998; Papadatou et al. 2002; Revicki, Whitley, and Gallery 1993; Wippen and Canellos 1991.
15. Steinhauser et al. 2000.
16. Arluke 2004b; Atwood-Harvey 2004; Crowell-Davis, Crowe, and Levine 1988; Hart and Hart 1987; Heath 1997; Herzog, Vore, and New 1989; Main 2006; Rollin 1987; C. Sanders 1995; Sawyer 1999; Schneider 1996.

17. Wippen and Canellos 1991.
18. Fogle and Abrahamson 1990.
19. Dickinson, Roof, and Roof 2010.
20. Becker et al. 1961; Hafferty 1991; Lella and Pawluch 1988; Merton, Reader, and Kendall 1957; Smith and Kleinman 1989.
21. Arluke 2004b; Arluke and Hafferty 1996.
22. Hafferty 1988; Wear 1989.
23. Bosk 1979; Iedema, Jorm, and Lum 2009.
24. Hafferty 1988.
25. Goffman 1959, 14.
26. Arluke 1977; Bosk 1979.
27. Iedema, Jorm, and Lum 2009.
28. Researchers found that new veterinary graduates struggled with these issues during the first few years of practice (Gelberg and Gelberg 2005; Routly et al. 2002; Strand, Zaparanick, and Brace 2005).
29. Cohen-Salter et al. 2004; Edney 1988; Herzog, Vore, and New 1989; Pilgram 2010; Tinga et al. 2001.
30. Gardner and Hini 2006; Gelberg and Gelberg 2005; Gray and Moffett 2010.
31. Heath, Lanyon, and Lynch-Blosse 1996; Pritchard 1988.
32. Liashenko, Oguz, and Brunnquell 2006.
33. Liashenko, Oguz, and Brunnquell 2006; Rollin 2006b; Tannenbaum 1993, 1995.
34. Self et al. 1991; Self et al. 1996.
35. Self, Pierce, and Shadduck 1994.
36. Rollin 2006b.
37. Bateman 2007; Coe, Adams, and Bonnett 2007; Gray and Moffett 2010; Klingborg and Klingborg 2007; Kogan et al. 2004; Kurtz 2006; Milani 1995; Pilgram 2010.
38. Aspegren 1999; Kurtz, Silverman, and Draper 2005; Roberts and Aruguete 2000.
39. Porter-Williamson et al. 2004.
40. Nogueira Borden et al. 2010.
41. Yedidia et al. 2003.
42. Latham and Morris 2007.
43. Mills 1997.
44. Hart and Mader 1992.
45. Butler, Williams, and Koll 2002; Tinga et al. 2001.
46. Martin and Taunton 2006; Williams, Butler, and Sontag 1999.
47. Surveys of veterinarians also show that they believe they provide important emotional support to clients (Pilgram 2010).
48. Brown and Silverman 1999; Heath, Lynch-Blosse, and Lanyon 1996b; Martin et al. 2004.
49. Butler, Williams, and Koll 2002; Martin et al. 2004; Pilgram 2010.
50. Mills 1997.
51. Coe, Adams, and Bonnett 2007; Fogelberg and Farnsworth 2009; Klingborg and Klingborg 2007.
52. Heath 2002.

53. Similar behavior was also found in Gauthier's (2001) study of occupational deviance in veterinary practice.

54. Festinger 1957.

55. Granfield and Koenig 2003; Stover 1989.

56. For a definition of *declawing* and examination of the issue, see Atwood-Harvey 2005.

57. For example, see Antelyes 1988; Birbeck 2006; Hannah 1985, 2002; Main 2006; Schneider 1996; and Tannenbaum 1985.

58. Becker et al. 1961; Bosk 1979; Fox 1979, 1989; Granfield and Koenig 1997, 2003; Hafferty 1991; Merton, Reader, and Kendall 1957; Mumford 1970.

59. Merton, Reader, and Kendall 1957.

60. Arluke 2004a.

CHAPTER 5

1. Stanford and Keto 1991.

2. Tannenbaum 1993.

3. Rollin 1986, 2003.

4. Surveys support the claim that, for many of today's veterinary students, the decision to study veterinary science is influenced mainly by a desire to work with animals and, for some, a love of animals (see Heath and Lanyon 1996; and Heath, Lynch-Blosse, and Lanyon 1996a).

5. Arluke 1994b; Arluke and Sanders 1996.

6. Lazarus 1999.

7. Folkman and Lazarus 1985.

8. Folkman 1984.

9. Hannah 1985, 666–667.

10. Frommer and Arluke 1999; White and Shawhan 1996.

11. Cahill 1999.

12. Wolkomir and Powers 2007, 160.

13. Fox 1989; Smith and Kleinman 1989.

14. Parsons 1951.

15. Fox 1979.

16. Becker et al. 1961; Conrad 1988; Fox 1979, 1989; Hafferty 1991; Mumford 1970.

17. Arluke and Hafferty 1996.

18. Arluke 2004b.

19. Capaldo 2004.

20. Clinton Sanders (1995) contemplates the creation of "personhood" as a social accomplishment, arguing that personhood "may be acquired or forfeited, given or taken away. It is a matter of social identity that determines how a being is treated, the rights and freedoms he/she/it possesses, and even whether and under what conditions the being is allowed to live" (210).

21. Lawler 1994; Meerabeau and Page 1998.

22. Lella and Pawluch 1988.

23. D. Jones 1985.

24. Crawley 2004.

25. C. Sanders 2010.

26. Coser 1960; Francis 1994.

27. Gordon 1983.

28. T. Sanders 2004.

29. C. Sanders 1994a, 162.

30. Coombs et al. 1993.

31. Ibid.

32. Ibid.

33. In her ethnographic study of sex workers, Teela Sanders (2004) also found humor important in establishing trust in the researcher-participant relationship.

34. Smith and Kleinman 1989, 64.

35. Astedt-Kurki and Liukkonen 1994; Coser 1960; Francis 1994; Haas 1977; Harries 1995; Mallett 1993; Tracy, Myers, and Scott 2006.

36. Smith and Kleinman 1989.

37. Pogrebin and Poole 1988.

38. Scott 2007.

39. Iedema, Jorm, and Lum 2009.

40. Anspach 1993.

41. Ashforth and Kreiner 1999.

42. Coombs et al. 1993; Gordon 1983.

43. Hochschild 1983.

44. T. Sanders 2004.

45. Coombs et al. 1993.

46. Smith and Kleinman 1989.

47. Becker et al. 1961; Fox 1979, 1989; Hafferty 1991; Mumford 1970; Smith and Kleinman 1989.

48. Granfield and Koenig 2003.

49. See Clinton Sanders's (1994a) discussion of problematic clients for a definition of *good* and *bad* clients.

50. Sean Wensley's 2008 article discusses the need for improving communication with clients who may be reluctant to permit euthanasia because of a strong human-animal bond.

51. Frommer and Arluke 1999.

52. Arluke 1994b; Williams and Mills 2000.

53. Arluke and Sanders 1996, 89.

54. Hart, Hart, and Mader 1990.

55. Arluke and Sanders 1996, 90.

56. Arluke 1994b.

57. Chiappetta-Swanson 2005.

58. Arluke 1994b; Frommer and Arluke 1999.

59. White and Shawhan 1996.

60. Joffe 1978, 119.

61. Hochschild 1983; Wolkomir and Powers 2007.

62. Chiappetta-Swanson 2005.

63. McNicholas and Collis 1995; Podrazik et al. 2000.

64. Manette 2004.

65. Hart and Hart 1987.

66. Hart, Hart, and Mader 1990.

67. Unsworth, Rogelberg, and Bonilla 2010.

68. White and Shawhan 1996.

69. Stewart 1999.

70. See Folkman 1982.

71. Folkman 1984.

72. Arluke 2004a, 1994a.

73. Arluke and Sanders 1996; C. Sanders 1995.

74. Manette 2004, 35.

75. Anspach 1993.

76. Christakis 1999.

77. White and Shawhan 1996.

78. Seymour 2001.

79. Zussman 1992.

80. Timmermans 2002.

81. Field and James 1993.

82. Gardner and Hini 2006; Phillips-Miller, Campbell, and Morrison 2000; Rollin 1987.

83. Gardner and Hini 2006; Phillips-Miller, Campbell, and Morrison 2000; Rollin 1987; Strand, Zaparanick, and Brace 2005.

84. Rollin 1987.

85. Gardner and Hini 2006; Rollin 1987.

86. Arluke 1994b; Baran et al. 2009; Reeve, Rogelberg, et al. 2005; Rohlf and Bennett 2005.

87. Fogle and Abrahamson 1990; Hart and Hart 1987; Rohlf and Bennett 2005; Rollin 1986, 1987; C. Sanders 1995.

88. Chang and Hart 1995.

89. C. Sanders 2010.

90. Arluke 2004a.

91. Reeve, Spitzmüller, et al. 2005.

CONCLUSION

1. Arluke and Sanders 1996.

2. Rollin 2006b; Tannenbaum 1995.

3. Rollin 2006b.

4. Carol Morgan and Michael McDonald (2007) note four major sources of ethical tension in moral dilemmas, and participants experienced all four: differences in beliefs regarding the importance of animals, differences in beliefs regarding responsibility to animals, differences in assessment of the interest of animals, and differences in the interpretation of their professional role.

5. Milani 2006a.

6. Livingston 2002.

7. Rollin 1986.

8. Rollin 2002, 2006b.

9. Sanders 1995.

10. Gauthier 2001.

11. Samuelson 1988, 134.

12. Tannenbaum 1995.

13. Carbone 2004, 117.

14. Gauthier 2001; Roth 1994.

15. This fact comes from the American Veterinary Medical Association's *Report on Veterinary Compensation* (2008b).

16. American Veterinary Medical Association 2003; National Commission on Veterinary Economic Issues 2000; Slater and Slater 2000.

17. For example, Abbott 1988; Dingwall and Lewis 1983; Parsons 1954.

18. Roth 1994.

19. Freidson 1970.

20. Freidson 1970, 92.

21. Freidson 1970, 107.

22. Zekoff and Felsted 2004, 35.

23. Rollin 2002.

24. Main 2006.

25. Main 2006; Morgan and McDonald 2007; Rollin 2002; Tannenbaum 1995; Yeates and Main 2010.

26. Hauser, Cushman, and Kamen 2006.

27. Lofflin 2004.

28. Charlton 1997.

29. Hankin 2007.

30. Lofflin 2004.

31. Hauser, Cushman, and Kamen 2006.

32. For just a couple of examples found in law journals debating the changing status of animals in the law and how it might influence veterinary practice, see Nunalee and Weedon 2004 in the journal *Animal Law* and Gregory 2010 in the journal *Family Law Quarterly*.

33. American Veterinary Medical Association 2008c.

34. Irvine and Vermilya 2010.

35. American Veterinary Medical Association 2008b; Bryant and Snizek 1985; S. Jones 2003.

36. S. Jones 2003.

37. Drum and Whiteley 1991; Lawrence 1997.

38. Phillips-Miller 2001; Zeglen 1980.

39. Slater and Slater 2000; Smith 2002.

40. Irvine and Vermilya 2010.

41. National Commission on Veterinary Economic Issues 2000; Slater and Slater 2000.

42. Morgan 2007; Rollin 2006a; Wojciechowska and Hewson 2005.

43. McGreevy and Dixon 2005.

44. Arkow 1994; Hymen 1995; Patronek 1997; Rollin 1994.

45. American Veterinary Medical Association 2008a.

46. For definition and examination of the issue of declawing, see Atwood-Harvey 2005.

47. American Veterinary Medical Association 2008a.

48. Antelyes 1988.

49. Arluke 2004b.

50. Capaldo 2004.

51. Dodge 1989; Hart and Wood 2004; McGreevy and Dixon 2005; Pritchard 1993; Scalese and Issenberg 2005; Schwartz 1990.

52. Lawrence 1997; National Commission on Veterinary Economic Issues 2000.

53. Pritchard 1993.

54. This term was also used by Clinton Sanders's (1994a) participants.

55. Lagoni, Hetts, and Butler 1994; Ormerod 2008.

56. Martin and Taunton 2006; Williams, Butler, and Sontag 1999.

APPENDIX

1. Glaser and Strauss 1967.

2. Berg 2004.

3. American Veterinary Medical Association 2008b.

4. American Veterinary Medical Association 2011; Chieffo, Kelly, and Ferguson 2008.

5. Lofland et al. 2005.

6. Shaffir and Stebbins 1991; Warren and Karner 2005.

7. T. Sanders 2004.

8. Francis 1994.

References

Abbott, Andrew. 1988. *The System of Professions*. Chicago: University of Chicago Press.

Abood, Sarah. 2008. "Effectively Communicating with Your Clients." *Topics in Companion Animal Medicine* 23 (3): 143–147.

Adams, Cindy, Brenda Bonnett, and Alan Meek. 2000. "Predictors of Owner Response to Companion Animal Death in 177 Clients from 14 Practices in Ontario." *Journal of the American Veterinary Medical Association* 217 (9): 1303–1309.

Albert, Alexa, and Kris Bulcroft. 1988. "Pets, Families, and the Life Course." *Journal of Marriage and the Family* 50 (2): 543–552.

American Veterinary Medical Association. 2001. "2000 Report of the American Veterinary Medical Association Panel on Euthanasia." *Journal of the American Medical Association* 218 (5): 669–692.

———. 2003. "Economic Report on Veterinarians and Veterinary Practices." Schaumburg, IL: Center for Information Management of the American Veterinary Medical Association.

———. 2007. "U.S. Pet Ownership and Demographics Sourcebook." Schaumburg, IL: Center for Information Management of the American Veterinary Medical Association.

———. 2008a. "Principles of Veterinary Medical Ethics of the AVMA." Schaumburg, IL: Center for Information Management of the American Veterinary Medical Association.

———. 2008b. "Report on Veterinary Compensation." Schaumburg, IL: Center for Information Management of the American Veterinary Medical Association.

———. 2008c. "Results of the 2006 AVMA Survey of Companion Animal Ownership in US Pet-Owning Households." *Journal of the American Veterinary Medical Association* 232 (5): 695–696.

———. 2011. "Market Research Statistics: U.S. Veterinarians—2010." AVMA, February. Available at http://www.avma.org/reference/marketstats/usvets.asp.

Anspach, Renee. 1993. *Deciding Who Lives: Fateful Choices in the Intensive Care Nursery.* Berkeley: University of California Press.

Antelyes, Jacob. 1988. "Convenience Euthanasia Revisited." *Journal of the American Veterinary Medical Association* 193 (8): 906–908.

————. 1991. "Conditions Requiring Chronic Management." *Problems in Veterinary Medicine* 3 (1): 51–60.

Archar, John, and George Winchester. 1994. "Bereavement following Death of a Pet." *British Journal of Psychology* 85 (part 2): 259–271.

Arkow, Phil. 1994. "Child Abuse, Animal Abuse, and the Veterinarian." *Journal of the American Veterinary Medical Association* 204 (7): 1004–1007.

Arluke, Arnold. 1977. "Social Control Rituals in Medicine: The Case of Death Rounds." In *Health Care and Health Knowledge*, edited by Robert Dingwall, Christian Heath, Margaret Reid, and Margaret Stacey, 107–125. New York: Prodist.

————. 1980. "Roundsmanship: Inherent Control on a Medical Teaching Ward." *Social Science and Medicine* 14A (4): 297–302.

————. 1988. "Sacrificial Symbolism in Animal Experimentation: Object or Pet?" *Anthrozoos* 2 (2): 98–117.

————. 1991a. "Coping with Euthanasia: A Case Study of Shelter Culture." *Journal of the American Medical Association* 198 (7): 1176–1180.

————. 1991b. "Going into the Closet with Science: Information Control among Animal Experimenters." *Journal of Contemporary Ethnography* 20 (3): 306–330.

————. 1994a. "The Ethical Socialization of Animal Researchers." *Lab Animal* 23 (6): 30–35.

————. 1994b. "Managing Emotions in an Animal Shelter." In *Animals and Human Society*, edited by Aubrey Manning and James Serpell, 145–165. New York: Routledge.

————. 1997. "Veterinary Education: A Plea and Plan for Sociological Study." *Anthrozoos* 10 (1): 3–7.

————. 2004a. *Brute Force: Animal Police and the Challenge of Cruelty.* West Lafayette, IN: Purdue University Press.

————. 2004b. "The Use of Dogs in Medical and Veterinary Training: Understanding and Approaching Student Uneasiness." *Journal of Applied Animal Welfare Science* 7 (3): 197–204.

Arluke, Arnold, and Frederic Hafferty. 1996. "From Apprehension to Fascination with 'Dog Lab': The Use of Absolutions by Medical Students." *Journal of Contemporary Ethnography* 25 (2): 191–209.

Arluke, Arnold, and Clinton Sanders. 1996. *Regarding Animals.* Philadelphia: Temple University Press.

Ashforth, Blake, and Glen Kreiner. 1999. "'How Can You Do It?': Dirty Work and the Challenge of Construction a Positive Identity." *Academy of Management Review* 24 (3): 413–434.

Aspegren, Knut. 1999. *Best Evidence Medical Education Guide 2: Teaching and Learning Communication Skills in Medicine: A Review with Quality Grading of Articles.* Dundee, UK: Association for Medical Education in Europe, Center for Medical Education.

Astedt-Kurki, Paivi, and Arja Liukkonen. 1994. "Humour in Nursing Care." *Journal of Advanced Nursing* 20 (1): 183–188.

Atwood-Harvey, Dana. 2004. "Interspecies Encounters: An Ethnography of a Veterinary Hospital." *Dissertation Abstracts International* 64, no. 7 (June): 2650-A.

————. 2005. "Death or Declaw: Dealing with Moral Ambiguity in a Veterinary Hospital." *Society and Animals* 13 (4): 315–342.

Baran, Benjamin, Joseph Allen, Steven Rogelberg, Christiane Spitzmüller, Natalie DiGiacomo, Jennifer Webb, Nathan Carter, Olga Clark, Lisa Teeter, and Alan Walker. 2009. "Euthanasia-Related Strain and Coping Strategies in Animal Shelter Employees." *Journal of the American Veterinary Medical Association* 235 (1): 83–88.

Barker, Sandra, and Randolph Barker. 1988. "The Human-Canine Bond: Closer Than Family Ties?" *Journal of Mental Health Counseling* 10 (1): 46–56.

Bateman, Shane. 2007. "Communication in the Veterinary Emergency Setting." *Veterinary Clinics of North America: Small Animal Practice* 37 (1): 109–121.

Beck, Alan, and Aaron Katcher. 1996. *Between Pets and People: The Importance of Animal Companionship.* West Lafayette, IN: Purdue University Press.

Becker, Howard, Blanche Geer, Everett Hughes, and Anselm Strauss. 1961. *Boys in White: Student Culture in Medical School.* Chicago: University of Chicago Press.

Belk, Russell. 1996. "Metamorphic Relationships with Pets." *Society and Animals* 4 (2): 121–145.

Berg, Bruce. 2004. *Qualitative Research Methods for the Social Sciences.* Boston: Allyn and Bacon.

Bilger, Burkhard. 2003. "The Last Meow: Organ Transplants, Chemotherapy, Root Canal: How Far Would You Go for a Pet?" *New Yorker*, September 8, pp. 46–53.

Birbeck, Tony. 2006. "Ethical Issues in the Provision of Veterinary Services." *Veterinary Record: Journal of the British Veterinary Association* 158 (4): 139–140.

Boles, Jacqueline, Phillip Davis, and Charlotte Tatro. 1983. "False Pretense and Deviant Exploitation: Fortunetelling as a Con." *Deviant Behavior* 4:375–394.

Bosk, Charles. 1979. *Forgive and Remember: Managing Medical Failure.* Chicago: University of Chicago Press.

Brabant, Sarah. 1997. "Guilt and Shame: Problematic Emotions in Grief Counseling." In *Social Perspectives on Emotion*, vol. 4, edited by David D. Franks, Beverley Cuthbertson-Johnson, and Rebecca Erickson, 103–124. Bingley, UK: Emerald Group.

Brissett, Dennis, and Charles Edgley. 1990. *Life as Theater: A Dramaturgical Sourcebook.* 2nd ed. New York: Aldine de Gruyter.

Brown, Bradford. 2006. *While You're Here, Doc: Farmyard Adventures of a Maine Veterinarian.* Gardiner, ME: Tilbury House.

Brown, Brenda, Herbert Richards, and Carol Wilson. 1996. "Pet Bonding and Pet Bereavement among Adolescents." *Journal of Counseling and Development* 74 (5): 505–509.

Brown, John, and Jon Silverman. 1999. "The Current and Future Market for Veterinarians and Veterinary Medical Services in the United States." *Journal of the American Veterinary Medical Association* 215 (2): 161–183.

Bryant, Clifton. 1979. "The Zoological Connection: Animal-Related Human Behavior." *Social Forces* 58 (2): 399–421.

Bryant, Clifton, and William Snizek. 1976. "Practice Modes and Professional Role Playing among Large and Small Animal Veterinarians." *Rural Sociology* 41 (2): 179–193.

————. 1985. "Animal Doctors: Careers, Clientele, and Practice Modes of Veterinarians." In *The Rural Work Force: Non-agricultural Occupations in America*, edited by

Clifton Bryant, Donald Shoemaker, James Skipper, and William Snizek, 199–217. South Hadley, MA: Bergin and Garvey.

Burghardt, Gordon, and Harold Herzog. 1989. "Attitudes toward Animals: Origins and Diversity." *Anthrozoos* 1 (4): 214–222.

Burrage, Michael. 1990. "The Professions in Sociology and History." In *Professions in Theory and History: Rethinking the Study of the Professions*, edited by Michael Burrage and Rolf Torstendahl, 1–23. London: Sage.

Bustad, Leo, Linda Hines, and Charles Leathers. 1981. "The Human–Companion Animal Bond and the Veterinarian." *Veterinary Clinics of North America: Small Animal Practice* 11 (4): 787–810.

Butler, Carolyn, Susan Williams, and Sharon Koll. 2002. "Perceptions of Fourth-Year Veterinary Students Regarding Emotional Support of Clients in Veterinary Practice in the Veterinary College Curriculum." *Journal of the American Veterinary Medical Association* 221 (3): 360–363.

Cahill, Spencer. 1999. "Emotional Capital and Professional Socialization: The Case of Mortuary Science Students (and Me)." *Social Psychology Quarterly* 62 (2): 101–116.

Cahill, Spencer, and Robin Eggleston. 1994. "Managing Emotions in Public: The Case of Wheelchair Users." *Social Psychology Quarterly* 57 (4): 300–312.

Cain, Ann. 1983. "A Study of Pets in the Family System." In *New Perspectives on Our Lives with Companion Animals*, edited by Aaron Katcher and Alan Beck, 72–81. Philadelphia: University of Pennsylvania Press.

Cameron, Alexander. 1990. *Poultry in the Pulpit: Further Revelations of the Vet in the Vestry*. New York: St. Martin's Press.

Capaldo, Theodora. 2004. "The Psychological Effects on Students of Using Animals in Ways that They See as Ethically, Morally or Religiously Wrong." *Alternatives to Laboratory Animals* 32 (1B): 525–531.

Carbone, Larry. 2004. "Centaurs and Science: The Professionalization of Laboratory Animal Care and Use." In *What Animals Want: Expertise and Advocacy in Laboratory Animal Welfare*, by Larry Carbone, 116–140. New York: Oxford University Press.

Carmack, Betty. 1985. "The Effects on Family Members and Functioning after the Death of Pet." In *Pets and the Family*, edited by Marvin B. Sussman, 149–162. New York: Haworth Press.

Case, Carole. 1991. *Down the Backstretch: Racing and the American Dream*. Philadelphia: Temple University Press.

Chang, Fon, and Lynette Hart. 1995. "Human-Animal Bonds in the Laboratory: How Animal Behavior Affects the Perspective of Caregivers." *Institute for Laboratory Animal Research Journal* 43 (1): 10–18.

Charlton, Anna. 1997. "The Killing of the Noah's Ark Shelter Cats: Such a Little Harm." *Animal Rights Commentary*, December 4.

Charmaz, Kathy. 1980. *The Social Reality of Death: Death in Contemporary America*. Reading, MA: Addison-Wesley.

Chiappetta-Swanson, Catherine. 2005. "Dignity and Dirty Work: Nurses' Experiences in Managing Genetic Termination for Fetal Anomaly." *Qualitative Sociology* 28 (1): 93–115.

Chieffo, Carla, Alan Kelly, and James Ferguson. 2008. "Trends in Gender, Employment, Salary, and Debt of Graduates of US Veterinary Medical Schools and Colleges." *Journal of the American Veterinary Medical Association* 233 (6): 910–917.

Christakis, Nicholas. 1999. *Death Foretold: Prophecy and Prognosis in Medical Care.* Chicago: University of Chicago Press.

Chun, Ruthanne, and Laura Garrett. 2007. "Communicating with Oncology Clients." *Veterinary Clinics of North America: Small Animal Practice* 37 (6): 1013–1022.

Chur-Hansen, Anna. 2010. "Grief and Bereavement Issues and the Loss of a Companion Animal: People Living with a Companion Animal, Owners of Livestock, and Animal Support Workers." *Clinical Psychologist* 14 (1): 14–21.

Clark, Candace. 1997. *Misery and Company: Sympathy in Everyday Life.* Chicago: University of Chicago Press.

Clark, Robert, and Emily LaBeff. 1982. "Death Telling: Managing the Delivery of Bad News." *Journal of Health and Social Behavior* 23 (4): 366–380.

Coates, Thomas J., and Bernard Lo. 1990. "Counseling Patients Seropositive for Human Immunodeficiency Virus: An Approach for Medical Practice." *Western Journal of Medicine* 153 (6): 629–634.

Coe, Jason, Cindy Adams, and Brenda Bonnett. 2007. "A Focus Group Study of Veterinarians' and Pet Owners' Perceptions of the Monetary Aspects of Veterinary Care." *Journal of the American Veterinary Medical Association* 231 (10): 1510–1518.

Cohen, Jonathan, Stephan Fihn, Edward Boyko, Albert Jonsen, and Robert Wood. 1994. "Attitudes toward Assisted Suicide and Euthanasia among Physicians in Washington State." *New England Journal of Medicine* 331 (2): 89–94.

Cohen, Susan. 2002a. "Can Pets Function as Family Members?" *Western Journal of Nursing Research* 24 (6): 621–638.

———. 2002b. "The Role of Social Work in a Veterinary Hospital Setting." *Veterinary Clinics of North America: Small Animal Practice* 15 (2): 355–363.

Cohen-Salter, Cynthia, Susan Folmer-Brown, Kimberly Hogrefe, Margaret Brosnahan. 2004. "A Model Euthanasia Workshop: One Class's Experience at Tufts University." *Journal of Veterinary Medical Education* 31 (1): 72–75.

Collins, Randall. 1990. "Market Closure and the Conflict Theory of the Professions." In *Professions in Theory and History: Rethinking the Study of the Professions*, edited by Michael Burrage and Rolf Torstendahl, 24–43. London: Sage.

Conrad, Peter. 1988. "Learning to Doctor: Reflections on Recent Accounts of the Medical School Years." *Journal of Health and Social Behavior* 29 (4): 323–332.

Coombs, Robert, Sangeeta Chopra, Debra Schenk, and Elaine Yutan. 1993. "Medical Slang and Its Functions." *Social Science and Medicine* 36 (8): 987–998.

Cornell, Karen, and Michelle Kopcha. 2007. "Client-Veterinarian Communication: Skills for Client Centered Dialogue and Shared Decision Making." *Veterinary Clinics of North America: Small Animal Practice* 37 (1): 37–47.

Coser, Rose Laub. 1960. "Laughter among Colleagues: A Study of the Functions of Humour among the Staff of a Mental Hospital." *Psychiatry* 23:81–95.

Crawley, Elaine. 2004. "Emotion and Performance: Prison Officers and the Presentation of Self in Prisons." *Punishment and Society* 6 (4): 411–427.

Croke, Vicki. 1999. *Animal ER: Extraordinary Stories of Hope and Healing from One of the World's Leading Veterinary Hospitals.* Harmondsworth, UK: Penguin Group.

Crowell-Davis, Sharon, Dennis Crowe, and David Levine. 1988. "Death and Euthanasia: Attitudes of Students and Faculty at a Veterinary Teaching Hospital." In *Euthanasia of the Companion Animal*, edited by William Kay, Susan Cohen,

Carole Fudin, Austin Kutscher, Herbert Neiburg, Ross Grey, and Mohamed Osman, 199–207. Philadelphia: Charles Press.

DeCoster, Vaughn A. 1997. "Physician Treatment of Patient Emotions: An Application of the Sociology of Emotion." In *Social Perspectives on Emotion*, edited by Rebecca Erickson and Beverley Cuthbertson-Johnson, 151–177. Greenwich, CT: JAI Press.

De Lorenzo, Robert, and James Augustine. 2004. "Lessons in Emergency Evacuation from the Miamisburg Train Derailment." *Prehospital Disaster Medicine* 11 (4): 270–275.

Dickinson, George, Paul Roof, and Karen Roof. 2010. "End-of-Life Issues in United States Veterinary Medicine Schools." *Society and Animals* 18 (2): 152–162.

Dingwall, Robert, and Philip Lewis. 1983. *The Sociology of the Professions: Lawyers, Doctors, and Others*. London: Macmillan Press.

Dodge, Susan. 1989. "Under Pressure from Students, Medical Schools Offer Alternatives to Use of Live Animals in Experiments." *Chronicle of Higher Education* November 15, pp. A41, A43.

Doherty, Nicole, and Judith Feeney. 2004. "The Composition of Attachment Networks throughout the Adult Years." *Personal Relationships* 11 (4): 469–488.

Doka, Kenneth. 2002. *Disenfranchised Grief: New Directions, Challenges, and Strategies for Practice*. Champaign, Illinois: Research Press.

Drum, Sue, and H. Ellen Whiteley. 1991. *Women in Veterinary Medicine: Profiles of Success*. Ames: Iowa State University Press.

Dunn, Kathleen, Stephen Mehler, and Helaine Greenberg. 2005. "Social Work with a Pet Loss Support Group in a University Veterinary Hospital." *Social Work in Health Care* 41 (2): 59–70.

Edney, Andrew. 1988. "Breaking the News: The Problems and Some Answers." In *Euthanasia of the Companion Animal*, edited by William Kay, Susan Cohen, Carole Fudin, Austin Kutscher, Herbert Neiburg, Ross Grey, and Mohamed Osman, 181–185. Philadelphia: Charles Press.

Emanuel, Ezekiel. 1994. "The History of Euthanasia Debates in the United States and Britain." *Annals of Internal Medicine* 121 (10): 793–802.

Etzioni, Amitai, ed. 1969. *The Semi-professions and Their Organization: Teachers, Nurses, Social Workers*. New York: Free Press.

Festinger, Leon. 1957. *A Theory of Cognitive Dissonance*. Stanford, CA: Stanford University Press.

Field, David. 1998. "Special Not Different: General Practitioners' Accounts of Their Care of Dying People." *Social Science Medicine* 46 (9): 111–120.

Field, David, and Nicky James. 1993. "Where and How People Die." In *The Future for Palliative Care: Issues of Policy and Practice*, edited by David Clark, 6–29. Buckingham, PA: Open University Press.

Field, Nigel, Lisa Orsini, Roni Gavish, and Wendy Packman. 2009. "Role of Attachment in Response to Pet Loss." *Death Studies* 33 (4): 334–355.

Fogelberg, Katherine, and Charles Farnsworth. 2009. "Faculty and Students' Self-Assessment of Client Communication Skills and Professional Ethics in Three Veterinary Medical Schools." *Journal of Veterinary Medical Education* 36 (4): 423–428.

Fogle, Bruce, and David Abrahamson. 1990. "Pet Loss: A Survey of the Attitudes and Feelings of Practicing Veterinarians." *Anthrozoos* 3 (3): 143–150.

Folkman, Susan. 1982. "An Approach to the Measurement of Coping." *Journal of Occupational Behavior* 3 (1): 95–107.

———. 1984. "Personal Control and Stress and Coping Processes: A Theoretical Analysis." *Journal of Personality and Social Psychology* 46 (4): 839–852.

Folkman, Susan, and Richard Lazarus. 1985. "If It Changes It Must Be a Process: Study of Emotion and Coping during Three Stages of a College Examination." *Journal of Personality and Social Psychology* 48 (1): 150–170.

Foster, Rory. 1985. *Dr. Wildlife: The Crusade of a Northwoods Vet.* New York: Watts.

Fox, Renee. 1979. *Essays in Medical Sociology: Journeys into the Field.* New York: Wiley.

———. 1989. *The Sociology of Medicine: A Participant Observer's View.* Englewood Cliffs, NJ: Prentice Hall.

Francis, Linda. 1994. "Laughter, the Best Mediation: Humor as Emotion Management in Interaction." *Symbolic Interaction* 17 (2): 147–163.

Francis, Linda, Kathleen Monahan, and Candyce Berger. 1999. "A Laughing Matter? The Use of Humor in Medical Interactions." *Motivation and Emotion* 23 (2): 155–174.

Franklin, Adrian. 1999. *Animals and Modern Cultures: A Sociology of Human-Animal Relations in Modernity.* London: Sage.

Freidson, Eliot. 1970. *The Profession of Medicine: A Study of the Sociology of Applied Knowledge.* Chicago: University of Chicago Press.

Friedman, Raymond. 1994. *Front Stage, Backstage: The Dramatic Structure of Labor Negotiations.* Cambridge, MA: MIT Press.

Friedman, Raymond, and Darren McDaniel. 1998. "In the Eye of the Beholder: Ethnography in the Study of Work." In *Researching the World of Work*, edited by Keith Wilson and George Barker, 113–126. Ithaca, NY: ILR Press.

Frommer, Stephanie, and Arnold Arluke. 1999. "Loving Them to Death: Blame-Displacing Strategies of Animal Shelter Workers and Surrenderers." *Society and Animals* 7 (1): 1–16.

Fuller, Ruth L., and Sally B. Geis. 1985. "Communicating with the Grieving Family." *Journal of Family Practice* 21 (2): 139–144.

Gage, Geraldine, and Ralph Holcomb. 1991. "Couples' Perception of Stressfulness of Death of the Family Pet." *Family Relations* 40 (1): 103–105.

Gage, Loretta, and Nancy Gage. 1994. *If Wishes Were Horses: The Education of a Veterinarian.* New York: St. Martin's Press.

Gardner, Dianne, and Dean Hini. 2006. "Work-Related Stress in the Veterinary Profession in New Zealand." *New Zealand Veterinary Journal* 54 (3): 119–124.

Gauthier, DeAnn. 2001. "Professional Lapses: Occupational Deviance and Neutralization Techniques in Veterinary Medical Practice." *Deviant Behavior* 22 (6): 467–490.

Gaylin, Willard, Leon Kass, Edmond Pelligrino, and Mark Siegler. 1988. "Doctors Must Not Kill." *Journal of the American Medical Association* 259 (14): 2139–2140.

Gelberg, Susan, and Howard Gelberg. 2005. "Stress Management Interventions for Veterinary Students." *Journal of Veterinary Medical Education* 32 (2): 173–181.

Gerwolls, Marilyn K., and Susan M. Labott. 1994. "Adjustment to the Death of a Companion Animal." *Anthrozoos* 7 (3): 172–187.

Gianelli, Diane. 1994. "Survey Yields Admissions of Doctor-Assisted Suicide." *American Medical News*, October 10, p. 6.

Glaser, Barney, and Anselm Strauss. 1965. *Awareness of Dying*. London: Weidenfeld and Nicolson.

———. 1967. *The Discovery of Grounded Theory: Strategies for Qualitative Research*. Piscataway, NJ: Aldine Transaction.

Godwin, Sandra. 2004. "Managing Guilt: The Personal Responsibility Rhetoric among Parents of 'Troubled' Teens." *Sociological Quarterly* 45 (3): 575–596.

Goffman, Erving. 1959. *The Presentation of Self in Everyday Life*. Garden City, New York: Anchor Books.

———. 1963. *Behavior in Public Places: Notes on the Social Organization of Gatherings*. New York: Free Press.

———. 1967. *Interaction Ritual: Essays on Face-to-Face Behavior*. Garden City, NY: Anchor Books.

Goodrum, Sarah, and Mark Stafford. 2003. "The Management of Emotions in the Criminal Justice System." *Sociological Focus* 36 (3): 179–196.

Gordon, David Paul. 1983. "Hospital Slang for Patients: Crocks, Gomers, Gorks and Others." *Language in Society* 12 (2): 173–185.

Gosse, Gerald H., and Michael J. Barnes. 1994. "Human Grief Resulting from the Death of a Pet." *Anthrozoos* 7 (2): 103–112.

Granfield, Robert, and Thomas Koenig. 1997. "Can Law School Idealism Survive? Implications for Progressive Lawyers." *Guild Practitioner* 54, no. 3 (Summer): 155–173.

———. 2003. "It's Hard to Be a Human Being and a Lawyer: Young Attorneys and the Confrontation with Ethical Ambiguity in Legal Practice." *West Virginia Law Review* 105, no. 2 (Winter): 495–524.

Gray, Carol, and Jenny Moffet. 2010. *Handbook of Veterinary Communication Skills*. Chichester, UK: Blackwell.

Greenberg, Samuel. 1997. *Euthanasia and Assisted Suicide: Psychosocial Issues*. Springfield, IL: Charles C. Thomas.

Greenebaum, Jessica. 2004. "It's a Dog's Life: Elevating Status from Pet to 'Fur Baby' at Yappy Hour." *Society and Animals* 12 (2): 117–135.

Gregory, John. 2010. "Pet Custody: Distorting Language and the Law." *Family Law Quarterly* 44 (1): 35–64.

Gregory, Stanford W., and Stephen Keto. 1991. "Creation of the 'Virtual Patient' in Medical Interaction: A Comparison of Doctor/Patient and Veterinarian/Client Relationships." Paper presented at the meeting of the American Sociological Association, August 23–27, Cincinnati, OH.

Grier, Katherine. 2006. *Pets in America: A History*. Orlando, FL: Harcourt Books.

Groves, James E. 1978. "Taking Care of the Hateful Patient." *New England Journal of Medicine* 298 (6): 883–887.

Guerrier, Yvonne, and Amel Adib. 2003. "Work at Leisure and Leisure at Work: A Study of the Emotional Labor of Tour Reps." *Human Relations* 56 (11): 1399–1417.

Haas, Jack. 1977. "Learning Real Feelings: A Study of High Steel Ironworkers' Reaction to Fear and Danger." *Sociology of Work and Occupations* 4 (2): 147–170.

Haas, Jack, and William Shaffir. 1977. "Taking on the Role of Doctor: A Dramaturgical Analysis of Professionalization." *Symbolic Interaction* 5 (2): 187–203.

———. 1982. "The Professionalization of Medical Students: Developing Competence and a Cloak of Competence." *Symbolic Interaction* 1 (1): 71–88.

Haddock, Sally, and Kathy Matthews. 1985. *The Making of a Woman Vet*. New York: Simon and Schuster.

Hafferty, Frederic. 1988. "Cadaver Stories and the Emotional Socialization of Medical Students." *Journal of Health and Social Behavior* 29 (4): 344–356.

———. 1991. *Into the Valley: Death and the Socialization of Medical Students*. New Haven, CT: Yale University Press.

Halliwell, Richard, and Brian Hoskin. 2005. "Reducing the Suicide Rate among Veterinary Surgeons: How the Profession Can Help." *Veterinary Record* 157 (14): 397–398.

Hankin, Susan. 2007. "Not a Living Room Sofa: Changing the Legal Status of Companion Animals." *Rutgers Journal of Law and Public Policy* 4 (2): 314–410.

Hannah, Harold. 1985. "Refusal to Treat and Refusal to Continue Treatment." *Journal of the American Veterinary Medical Association* 186 (7): 666–668.

———. 2002. "The Ethical Content of Veterinary Medical Practice Acts." *Journal of the American Veterinary Medical Association* 220 (5): 610–611.

Harries, Gill. 1995. "Use of Humour in Patient Care." *British Journal of Nursing* 4 (17): 984–986.

Hart, Lynette, and Benjamin Hart. 1987. "Grief and Stress from So Many Animal Deaths." *Companion Animal Practice* 1:20–21.

Hart, Lynette, Benjamin Hart, and Bonnie Mader. 1990. "Humane Euthanasia and Companion Animal Death: Caring for the Animal, the Client, and the Veterinarian." *Journal of the American Veterinary Medical Association* 197 (10): 1292–1299.

Hart, Lynette, and Bonnie Mader. 1992. "Pet Loss Support Hotline: The Veterinary Students' Perspective." *California Veterinarian* 46 (1): 19–22.

Hart, Lynette, and Mary Wood. 2004. "Uses of Animals and Alternatives in College and Veterinary Education at the University of California, Davis: Institutional Commitment for Mainstreaming Alternatives." *Alternatives to Laboratory Animals* 32 (1): 617–620.

Hauser, Marc, Fiery Cushman, and Matthew Kamen. 2006. *People, Property or Pets?* West Lafayette, IN: Purdue University Press.

Heath, Sebastian, Philip Kass, Alan Beck and Larry Glickman. 2001. "Human and Pet-Related Risk Factors for Household Evacuation Failure during a Natural Disaster." *American Journal of Epidemiology* 153 (7): 659–665.

Heath, Trevor. 1997. "Experiences and Attitudes of Recent Veterinary Graduates: A National Survey." *Australian Veterinary Practice* 27 (1): 45–50.

———. 2002. "Longitudinal Study of Veterinarians from Entry to the Veterinary Course to 10 Years after Graduation: Attitudes to Work, Career and Profession." *Australian Veterinary Journal* 80 (8): 474–478.

Heath, Trevor, and Andrea Lanyon. 1996. "A Longitudinal Study of Veterinary Students and Recent Graduates: Gender Issues." *Australian Veterinary Journal* 74 (4): 305–308.

Heath, Trevor, Andrea Lanyon, and Mark Lynch-Blosse. 1996. "A Longitudinal Study of Veterinary Students and Recent Graduates: Perceptions of Veterinary Education." *Australian Veterinary Journal* 74 (4): 301–304.

Heath, Trevor, Mark Lynch-Blosse, and Andrea Lanyon. 1996a. "A Longitudinal Study of Veterinary Students and Recent Graduates: Backgrounds, Plans and Subsequent Employment." *Australian Veterinary Journal* 74 (4): 291–296.

———. 1996b. "A Longitudinal Study of Veterinary Students and Recent Graduates: Views of the Veterinary Profession." *Australian Veterinary Journal* 74 (4): 297–300.

Henry, Vincent. 2004. *Death Work: Police, Trauma, and the Psychology of Survival.* Oxford: Oxford University Press.

Herriot, James. 1972. *All Creatures Great and Small.* New York: St. Martin's Press.

Herzog, Hal. 2010. *Some We Love, Some We Hate, Some We Eat: Why It's So Hard to Think Straight about Animals.* New York: HarperCollins.

Herzog, Harold. 1993. "Human Morality and Animal Research." *American Scholar* 62:337–349.

Herzog, Harold, Tamara Vore, and John New. 1989. "Conversations with Veterinary Students: Attitudes, Ethics, and Animals." *Anthrozoos* 2 (3): 181–188.

Hetts, Suzanne, and Laurel Lagoni. 1990. "The Owner of the Pet with Cancer." *Veterinary Clinics of North America: Small Animal Practice* 20 (4): 879–896.

Hochschild, Arlie. 1979. "Emotion Work, Feeling Rules, and Social Structure." *American Journal of Sociology* 85 (3): 551–575.

———. 1983. *The Managed Heart.* Berkeley: University of California Press.

———. 1989. *The Second Shift.* New York: Avon.

Holloway, Jennifer. 2003. "Talking Dollars." *Money Matters* 1 (1): 1–2.

Holyfield, Lori, and Gary Allan Fine. 1997. "Adventure as Character Work: The Collective Taming of Fear." *Symbolic Interaction* 20 (4): 343–363.

Howarth, Glennys. 1996. *Last Rites: The Work of the Modern Funeral Director.* Amityville, NY: Baywood.

Humphry, Derek. 2002. *Final Exit: The Practicalities of Self-Deliverance and Assisted Suicide for the Dying.* 3rd ed. New York: Random House.

Hyland, Liam, and Janice Morse. 1995. "Orchestrating Comfort: The Role of Funeral Directors." *Death Studies* 19 (5): 453–474.

Hymen, Allen. 1995. "Laws Mandating Reporting of Domestic Violence: Do They Promote Patient Well-Being?" *Journal of the American Medical Association* 273 (22): 1781–1787.

Iedema, Rick, Christine Jorm, and Martin Lum. 2009. "Affect Is Central to Patient Safety: The Horror Stories of Young Anaesthetists." *Social Science and Medicine* 69 (12): 1750–1756.

Irvine, Leslie. 2004. *If You Tame Me: Understanding Our Connection with Animals.* Philadelphia: Temple University Press.

Irvine, Leslie, and Jenny Vermilya. 2010. "Gender Work in a Feminized Profession: The Case of Veterinary Medicine." *Gender and Society* 24 (1): 56–82.

Jesilow, Paul, Henry Pontell, and Gilbert Geis. 1993. *Prescription for Profit: How Doctors Defraud Medicare.* Berkeley: University of California Press.

Joffe, Carole. 1978. "What Abortion Counselors Want from Their Clients." *Social Problems* 26 (1): 112–121.

Jones, David. 1985. "Secondary Disaster Victims: The Emotional Effects of Recovering and Identifying Human Remains." *American Journal of Psychiatry* 142 (3): 303–307.

Jones, Lynn Cerys. 1997. "Both Friend and Stranger: How Crisis Volunteers Build and Manage Unpersonal Relationships with Clients." In *Social Perspectives on Emotion*, edited by Rebecca Erickson and Beverley Cuthbertson-Johnson, 125–148. Greenwich, CT: JAI Press.

Jones, Susan. 2003. *Valuing Animals: Veterinarians and Their Patients in Modern America*. Baltimore: Johns Hopkins University Press.

Kahler, Susan. 1992. "Stalking a Killer: The 'Disease' of Euthanasia." *Journal of the American Veterinary Medical Association* 201 (7): 973–975.

Katcher, Aaron. 1989. "How Companion Animals Make Us Feel." In *Perceptions of Animals in American Culture*, edited by R. Hoage, 113–127. Washington, DC: Smithsonian Institution Press.

Kearl, Michael. 1989. *Endings: A Sociology of Death and Dying*. New York: Oxford University Press.

Kellehear, Allan, and Jan Fook. 1997. "Lassie Come Home: A Study of 'Lost Pet' Notices." *Omega—Journal of Death and Dying* 34 (3): 191–202.

Kevorkian, Jack. 1991. *Prescription Medicide: The Goodness of Planned Death*. New York: Prometheus Books.

Kilarski, Barbara. 2003. "Keep Chickens! Tending Small Flocks in Cities, Suburbs, and Other Small Spaces." North Adams, MA: Storey.

Klingborg, Donald, and Jon Klingborg. 2007. "Talking with Veterinary Clients about Money." *Veterinary Clinics of North America: Small Animal Practice* 37 (1): 79–93.

Kogan, Lori, Carolyn Butler, Laurel Lagoni, Julia Brannan, Sherry McConnell, and Ashley Harvey. 2004. "Training in Client Relations and Communication Skills in Veterinary Medical Curricula and Usage after Graduation." *Journal of the American Veterinary Medical Association* 224 (4): 504–507.

Korczynski, Marek. 2003. "Communities of Coping: Collective Emotional Labor in Service Work." *Organization* 10 (1): 55–79.

Kurdek, Lawrence. 2008. "Pet Dogs as Attachment Figures." *Journal of Social and Personal Relationships* 25 (2): 247–266.

———. 2009. "Pet Dogs as Attachment Figures for Adult Owners." *Journal of Family Psychology* 23 (4): 439–446.

Kurtz, Suzanne. 2006. "Teaching and Learning Communication in Veterinary Medicine." *Journal of Veterinary Medical Education* 33 (1): 11–19.

Kurtz, Suzanne, Jonathan Silverman, and Juliet Draper. 2005. *Teaching and Learning Communication Skills in Medicine*. 2nd ed. Abingdon, UK: Radcliffe.

Lagoni, Laurel, Suzanne Hetts, and Carolyn Butler. 1994. *The Human-Animal Bond and Grief*. Philadelphia: Saunders.

Larson, Eric, and Xin Yao. 2005. "Clinical Empathy as Emotional Labor in the Patient-Physician Relationship." *Journal of the American Medical Association* 293 (9): 310–315.

Latham, Christine, and Arianwen Morris. 2007. "Effects of Formal Training in Communication Skills on the Ability of Veterinary Students to Communicate with Clients." *Veterinary Record* 160 (6): 181–186.

Lawler, Jocalyn. 1994. *Behind the Scenes: Nursing, Somology and the Problems of the Body*. Melbourne, Australia: Churchill Livingstone.

Lawrence, Elizabeth Atwood. 1988. "Those Who Dislike Pets." *Anthrozoos* 1 (3): 147–148.

———. 1997. "A Woman Veterinary Student in the Fifties: The View from the Approaching Millennium." *Anthrozoos* 10 (4): 160–169.

Lazarus, Richard. 1999. *Stress and Emotion: A New Synthesis*. London: Free Association Books.

Lee, Melinda, Heidi Nelson, Virginia Tilden, Linda Ganzini, Terri Schmidt, and Susan Tolle. 1996. "Legalizing Assisted Suicide—Views of Physicians in Oregon." *New England Journal of Medicine* 334 (5): 310–315.

Leif, Harold, and Renee Fox. 1963. "Training for 'Detached Concern' in Medical Students." In *The Psychological Basis of Medical Practice*, edited by Harold Leif, 12–35. New York: Harper and Row.

Lella, Joseph, and Dorothy Pawluch. 1988. "Medical Students and the Cadaver in Social and Cultural Context." In *Biomedicine Examined*, edited by Margaret Lock and Deborah Gordon, 125–154. New York: Kluwer Academic.

Lewis, Patricia. 2005. "Suppression of Expression: An Exploration of Emotion Management in a Special Care Baby Unit." *Work, Employment and Society* 19 (3): 565–581.

Liashenko, Joan, N. Yasemin Oguz, and Donald Brunnquell. 2006. "Critique of the 'Tragic Case' Methods in Ethics Education." *Journal of Medical Ethics* 32 (11): 672–677.

Livingston, Alexander. 2002. "Ethical Issues Regarding Pain in Animals." *Journal of the American Veterinary Medical Association* 221 (2): 229–233.

Lofflin, John. 2004. "The Changing Status of Pets." *Veterinary Economics*, February, pp. 32–38.

Lofland, John, David Snow, Leon Anderson, and Lyn Lofland. 2005. *Analyzing Social Settings: A Guide to Qualitative Observation and Analysis.* 4th ed. Belmont, CA: Wadsworth.

Lofland, Lyn. 1985. "The Social Shaping of Emotion: The Case of Grief." *Symbolic Interaction* 8 (2): 171–190.

Lois, Jennifer. 2001. "Managing Emotions, Intimacy, and Relationships in a Volunteer Search and Rescue Group." *Journal of Contemporary Ethnography* 30 (2): 131–179.

Lose, M. Phyllis. 1979. *No Job for a Lady: The Autobiography of M. Phyllis Lose.* New York: Macmillan.

Lowe, Sarah, Jean Rhodes, Liza Zwiebach, and Christian Chan. 2009. "The Impact of Pet Loss on the Perceived Social Support and Psychological Distress of Hurricane Survivors." *Journal of Traumatic Stress* 22 (3): 244–247.

MacDonald, Keith. 1995. *The Sociology of the Professions.* London: Sage.

Main, David. 2006. "Offering the Best to Patients: Ethical Issues Associated with the Provision of Veterinary Services." *Veterinary Record* 158 (2): 62–66.

Mallery, Kevin, Lisa Freeman, Neil Harpster, and John Rush. 1999. "Factors Contributing to the Decision for Euthanasia of Dogs with Congestive Heart Failure." *Journal of the American Veterinary Medical Association* 214 (8): 1201–1204.

Mallett, Jane. 1993. "Use of Humour and Laughter in Patient Care." *British Journal of Nursing* 2 (3): 172–175.

Manette, Cydria. 2004. "A Reflection on the Ways Veterinarians Cope with the Death, Euthanasia, and Slaughter of Animals." *Journal of the American Veterinary Medical Association* 225 (1): 34–38.

Manning, Aubrey, and James Serpell. 1994. *Animals and Human Society: Changing Perspectives.* London: Routledge.

Manning, Peter K. 1982. "Producing Drama: Symbolic Communication and the Police." *Symbolic Interaction* 5 (2): 223–241.

Martin, E. Alec. 2006. "Managing Client Communication for Effective Practice: What Skills Should Veterinary Graduates Have Acquired for Success?" *Journal of Veterinary Medical Education* 33 (1): 45–49.

Martin, Francois, Kathleen Ruby, Tiffany Deking, and Anne Taunton. 2004. "Factors Associated with Client, Staff, and Student Satisfaction regarding Small Animal Euthanasia Procedures at a Veterinary Teaching Hospital." *Journal of the American Veterinary Medical Association* 224 (11): 1774–1779.

Martin, Francois, and Anne Taunton. 2006. "Perceived Importance and Integration of the Human-Animal Bond in Private Veterinary Practice." *Journal of the American Veterinary Medical Association* 228 (4): 522–527.

McGreevy, Paul, and Robert Dixon. 2005. "Teaching Animal Welfare at the University of Sydney's Faculty of Veterinary Science." *Journal of Veterinary Medical Education* 32 (4): 442–446.

McNicholas, June, and Glyn Collis. 1995. "The End of a Relationship: Coping with Pet Loss." In *The WALTHAM Book of Human-Animal Interaction: Benefits and Responsibilities of Pet Ownership*, edited by I. Robinson, 127–143. Oxford: Pergamon, Elsevier Science.

Meerabeau, Liz, and Susie Page. 1998. "Getting the Job Done: Emotion Management and Cardiopulmonary Resuscitation in Nursing." In *Emotions in Social Life: Critical Themes and Contemporary Issues*, edited by Simon Williams, 291–312. London: Routledge.

Mercer, Laura. 2007. "Vet Social Work Program Counsels Pet Owners, Staff." *New Social Worker* 14 (2): 8.

Merton, Robert, George Reader, and Patricia Kendall. 1957. *The Student-Physician: Introductory Studies in the Sociology of Medical Education*. Cambridge, MA: Harvard University Press.

Meyers, Barbara. 2002. "Disenfranchised Grief and the Loss of an Animal Companion." In *Disenfranchised Grief: New Directions, Challenges, and Strategies for Practice*, edited by Kenneth Doka, 251–264. Champaign, IL: Research Press.

Milani, Myrna. 1995. *The Art of Veterinary Practice: A Guide to Client Communication*. Philadelphia: University of Pennsylvania Press.

———. 2004. "Practitioner-Client Communication: When Goals Conflict." *Canadian Veterinary Journal* 44 (8): 675–678.

———. 2006a. "Gender-Specific Animal References: Anthropomorphic Pandering or Quality Client Communication?" *Canadian Veterinary Journal* 47 (2): 171–174.

———. 2006b. "Problematic Client-Animal Relationships: The Analyzers." *Canadian Veterinary Journal* 47 (8): 813–816.

———. 2006c. "Problematic Client-Veterinarian Relationships: The 'Yes, Buts.'" *Canadian Veterinary Journal* 47 (10): 1025–1028.

Mills, Jennifer. 1997. "Use of Drama in Teaching the Human Side of Veterinary Practice." *Australian Veterinary Journal* 75 (7): 497–499.

Mizrahi, Terry. 1984. "Coping with Patients: Subcultural Adjustments to the Conditions of Work among Internists-in-Training." *Social Problems* 32 (2): 156–166.

———. 1986. *Getting Rid of Patients: Contradictions in the Socialization of Physicians*. New Brunswick, NJ: Rutgers University Press.

Morgan, Carol. 2007. "Autonomy and Paternalism in Quality of Life Determination in Veterinary Practice." *Animal Welfare* 16 (supp. 1): 143–147.

Morgan, Carol, and Michael McDonald. 2007. "Ethical Dilemmas in Veterinary Medicine." *Veterinary Clinics of North America: Small Animal Practice* 37 (1): 165–179.

Morley, Christine, and Jan Fook. 2005. "The Importance of Pet Loss and Some Implications for Services." *Mortality* 10 (2): 127–143.

Mumford, Emily. 1970. *Interns: From Students to Physicians.* Cambridge, MA: Harvard
University Press.

National Commission on Veterinary Economic Issues. 2000. "Current and Future Market
for Veterinarians and Veterinary Medical Services in the US." Schaumburg, IL: Center for Information Management of the American Veterinary Medical Association.

Nelson, Carnot, Ann Kurtz, and Geoffrey Hacker. 1988. "Hurricane Evacuation Behavior: Lessons from Elena." *Public Affairs Reporter* 2 (2): 1–3.

Nelson, Douglas. 1992. "Humor in the Pediatric Emergency Department: A 20-Year
Retrospective." *Pediatrics* 89 (6): 1089–1091.

Newfield, Susan, Neal Newfield, Jeannie Sperry, and Thomas Edward Smith. 2000.
"Ethical Decision Making among Family Therapist and Individual Therapists."
Family Process 39 (2): 177–188.

Nogueira Borden, Leandra, Cindy Adams, Brenda Bonnett, Jane Shaw, and Carl Rib-
ble. 2010. "Use of the Measure of Patient-Centered Communication to Analyze
Euthanasia Discussions in Companion Animal Practice." *Journal of the American
Veterinary Medical Association* 237 (11): 1275–1285.

Nunalee, Mary Margaret McEachern, and G. Robert Weedon. 2004. "Modern Trends
in Veterinary Malpractice: How Our Evolving Attitudes toward Nonhuman Animals Will Change Veterinary Medicine." *Animal Law* 10:125–161.

Nyman, Dag, Leonid Eidelman, and Charles Sprung. 1996. "Euthanasia." *Critical Care
Clinics* 12 (1): 85–96.

O'Kelley, Joyce. 1979. "Client Education through Friendly Persuasion." *Modern Veterinary Practice* 60 (1): 14–15.

Ormerod, Elizabeth. 2008. "Bond-Centered Veterinary Practice: Lessons for Veterinary
Faculty and Students." *Journal of Veterinary Medical Education* 35 (4): 545–552.

Palmer, Eddie, Sheryl Gonoulin, Ray Bias, and Wanda Eaves. 1992. "Financial Triage:
Strain, Stress, and Adaptation within Today's Medical System." *Prehospital and Disaster Medicine* 7:295–300.

Papadatou, Danai, Thalia Bellali, Irene Papazoglou, and Dimitra Petraki. 2002. "Greek
Nurse and Doctor Grief as a Result of Caring for Children Dying of Cancer." *Pediatric Nursing* 28 (4): 345–353.

Parsons, Talcott. 1951. *The Social System.* New York: Free Press.

———. 1954. "Professions and Social Structure." In *Essays in Sociological Theory,* 34–
49. Glencoe, IL: Free Press.

Pasko, Lisa. 2002. "Naked Power: The Practice of Stripping as a Confidence Game."
Sexualities 5 (1): 49–66.

Patronek, Gary. 1997. "Issues for Veterinarians in Recognizing and Reporting Animal
Neglect and Abuse." *Society and Animals* 5 (3): 267–280.

Phillips, Mary T. 1993. "Savages, Drunks, and Lab Animals: The Researcher's Perception of Pain." *Society and Animals* 1 (1): 61–82.

———. 1994. "Proper Names and the Social Construction of Biography: The Negative
Case of Laboratory Animals." *Qualitative Sociology* 17 (2): 119–142.

Phillips-Miller, Dianne. 2001. "Same Profession, Different Career: A Study of Men and
Women in Veterinary Medicine." In *Advances in Psychology Research,* vol. 5, edited
by Frank Columbus, 1–53. Hauppauge, NY: Nova Science.

Phillips-Miller, Dianne, N. Jo Campbell, and Charles Morrison. 2000. "Work and Family: Satisfaction, Stress, and Spousal Support." *Journal of Employment Counseling* 37 (1): 16–30.

Pilgram, Mary. 2010. "Communicating Social Support to Grieving Clients: The Veterinarian's View." *Death Studies* 34 (8): 699–714.

Planchon, Lynn A., and Donald I. Templer. 1996. "The Correlates of Grief after Death of a Pet." *Anthrozoos* 9 (2–3): 107–113.

Podrazik, Donna, Shane Shackford, Louis Becker, and Troy Heckert. 2000. "The Death of a Pet: Implications for Loss and Bereavement across the Lifespan." *Journal of Personal and Interpersonal Loss* 5 (4): 361–395.

Pogrebin, Mark, and Eric Poole. 1988. "Humor in the Briefing Room: A Study of the Strategic Uses of Humor among Police." *Symbolic Interaction* 17 (2): 147–163.

Porter-Williamson, Karin, Charles von Gunten, Karen Garman, Laurel Herbst, Harry Bluestein, and Wendy Evans. 2004. "Improving Knowledge in Palliative Medicine with a Required Hospice Rotation for Third-Year Medical Students." *Academic Medicine* 79 (8): 777–782.

Pritchard, William. 1988. "Future Directions for Veterinary Medicine." Durham, NC: Pew National Veterinary Education Program, Institute of Policy Sciences and Public Affairs.

———. 1993. "Comments on the Evolution of Veterinary Medical Education in the U.S. and Canada: Some Lessons from History." *Journal of Veterinary Medical Education* 20 (2): 53–55.

Ptacek, John, Karen Leonard, and Tara McKee. 2004. "'I've Got Some Bad News . . .': Veterinarians' Recollections of Communicating Bad News to Clients." *Journal of Applied Social Psychology* 34 (2): 366–390.

Quackenbush, James. 1985. "The Death of a Pet: How It Can Affect an Owner." *Veterinary Clinics of North America: Small Animal Practice* 15:395–402.

Rafaeli, Anat, and Robert Sutton. 1991. "Emotional Contrast Strategies as Means of Social Influence: Lessons from Criminal Interrogators and Bill Collectors." *Academy of Management Journal* 34 (4): 749–775.

Redinbaugh, Ellen, Amy Sullivan, Susan Block, Nina Gadmer, Matthew Lakoma, Ann Mitchell, Deborah Seltzer, Jennifer Wolford, and Robert Arnold. 2003. "Doctors' Emotional Reactions to Recent Death of a Patient: Cross Sectional Study of Hospital Doctors." *British Medical Journal* 327 (7408): 185–189.

Reeve, Charlie, Steven Rogelberg, Christine Spitzmüller, and Natalie DiGiacomo. 2005. "The Caring-Killing Paradox: Euthanasia-Related Strain among Animal-Shelter Workers." *Journal of Applied Social Psychology* 35 (1): 119–143.

Reeve, Charlie, Christine Spitzmüller, Steven Rogelberg, Alan Walker, Lisa Schultz, and Olga Clark. 2004. "Employee Reactions and Adjustment to Euthanasia-Related Work: Identifying Turning-Point Events through Retrospective Narratives." *Journal of Applied Animal Welfare Science* 7 (1): 1–25.

Revicki, Dennis, Theodore Whitley, and Michael Gallery. 1993. "Organizational Characteristics, Perceived Work Stress, and Depression in Emergency Medicine Residents." *Journal of Behavioral Medicine* 19 (2): 74–81.

Roberts, Alison, and Keri Smith. 2002. "Managing Emotions in the College Classroom: The Cultural Diversity Course as an Example." *Teaching Sociology* 30 (3): 291–303.

Roberts, Carlos, and Mara Aruguete. 2000. "Task and Socioemotional Behaviors of Physicians: A Test of Reciprocity and Social Interaction Theories in Analogue Physician-Patient Encounters." *Social Science and Medicine* 50 (3): 309–315.

Roberts, Felicia. 2004. "Speaking to and for Animals in a Veterinary Clinic: A Practice for Managing Interpersonal Interaction." *Research on Language and Social Interaction* 37 (4): 421–446.

Rohlf, Vanessa, and Pauleen Bennett. 2005. "Perpetration-Induced Traumatic Stress in Persons Who Euthanize Nonhuman Animals in Surgeries, Animal Shelters, and Laboratories." *Society and Animals* 13 (3): 201–219.

Rollin, Bernard. 1986. "Euthanasia and Moral Stress." *Loss, Grief and Care* 1 (1–2): 115–126.

———. 1994. "An Ethicist's Commentary on Whether Veterinarians Should Report Cruelty." *Canadian Veterinary Journal* 35 (7): 408–409.

———. 1999. *An Introduction to Veterinary Medical Ethics: Theory and Cases.* Ames: Iowa State University Press.

———. 2002. "The Use and Abuse of Aesculapian Authority in Veterinary Medicine." *Journal of the American Veterinary Medical Association* 220 (8): 1144–1149.

———. 2003. "An Ethicist's Commentary on Veterinarians Treating Unowned Animals and Euthanizing Unwanted Animals." *Canadian Veterinary Journal* 44 (5): 363–364.

———. 2006a. "Euthanasia and Quality of Life." *Journal of the American Veterinary Medical Association* 228 (7): 1014–1016.

———. 2006b. *An Introduction to Veterinary Medical Ethics: Theory and Cases.* 2nd ed. Ames: Iowa State University Press.

Ross, Cheri, and Jane Baron-Sorenson. 1998. *Pet Loss and Human Emotion: Guiding Clients through Grief.* Philadelphia: Accelerated Development.

Roth, Julius. 1994. *Animal Health Care: An Observational Study of the Practice of Veterinary Medicine.* University of California, Davis: Published by author.

Routly, J., I. Taylor, R. Turner, E. McKernan, and H. Dobson. 2002. "Support Needs of Veterinary Surgeons during the First Few Years of Practice: Perceptions of Recent Graduates and Senior Partners." *Veterinary Record* 150 (6): 167–171.

Rowe, Alison, and Cheryl Regehr. 2010. "Whatever Gets You through Today: An Examination of Cynical Humor among Emergency Service Professionals." *Journal of Loss and Trauma* 15:448–464.

Samuelson, Marvin. 1988. "Attitudes toward Animals and Their Effect on Veterinary Practice Management." In *Euthanasia of the Companion Animal,* edited by William Kay, Susan Cohen, Carole Fudin, Austin Kutscher, Herbert Neiburg, Ross Grey, and Mohamed Osman, 133–137. Philadelphia: Charles Press.

Sanders, Clinton. 1994a. "Annoying Owners: Routine Interactions with Problematic Clients in a General Veterinary Practice." *Qualitative Sociology* 17 (2): 159–170.

———. 1994b. "Biting the Hand that Heals You: Encounters with Problematic Patients in a General Veterinary Practice." *Society and Animals* 2 (1): 47–66.

———. 1995. "Killing with Kindness: Veterinary Euthanasia and the Social Construction of Personhood." *Sociological Forum* 10 (2): 195–214.

———. 1999. *Understanding Dogs: Living and Working with Canine Companions.* Philadelphia: Temple University Press.

————. 2010. "Working Out Back: The Veterinary Technician and 'Dirty Work.'" *Journal of Contemporary Ethnography* 39 (3): 243–272.

Sanders, Teela. 2004. "Controllable Laughter: Managing Sex Work through Humour." *Sociology* 38 (2): 273–291.

Sawicki, Stephen. 1996. *Animal Hospital*. Chicago: Chicago Review Press.

Sawyer, Marcia. 1999. "An Exploration of Ethical Dilemmas Experienced by Veterinary Medical Students in Their Clinical Training." Ph.D. diss., Cornell University.

Sayre, Joan. 2001. "The Use of Aberrant Medical Humor by Psychiatric Unit Staff." *Issues in Mental Health Nursing* 22 (7): 669–689.

Scalese, Ross, and Barry Issenberg. 2005. "Effective Use of Simulations for the Teaching and Acquisition of Veterinary Professional and Clinical Skills." *Journal of Veterinary Medical Association* 32 (4): 461–467.

Schneider, Beverley. 1996. "Euthanasia and the Veterinarian." *Canadian Veterinary Journal* 37 (4): 217–218.

Schoen, Allen. 1991. "Decision-Making Concerning Pets with Loss of Autonomic Function." *Problems in Veterinary Medicine* 3 (1): 61–72.

Schulman-Green, Dena. 2003. "Coping Mechanisms of Physicians Who Routinely Work with Dying Patients." *Omega—Journal of Death and Dying* 47 (3): 253–264.

Schwartz, Anthony. 1990. "Some Comments on 'Changing Social Ethics on Animals and Veterinary Medical Education.'" *Journal of Veterinary Medical Education* 17 (1): 6–7.

Scott, Tricia. 2007. "Expression of Humour by Emergency Personnel Involved in Sudden Deathwork." *Mortality* 12 (4): 350–364.

Seale, Clive. 2009. "Legalisation of Euthanasia or Physician-Assisted Suicide: Survey of Doctors' Attitudes." *Palliative Medicine* 203 (3): 205–212.

Self, Donnie, Nancy Jecker, DeWitt Baldwin, and John Shadduck. 1991. "Moral Orientations of Justice and Care among Veterinarians Entering Veterinary Practice." *Journal of the American Veterinary Medical Association* 199 (5): 569–573.

Self, Donnie, Margie Olivarez, DeWitt Baldwin, and John Shadduck. 1996. "Clarifying the Relationship of Veterinary Medical Education and Moral Development." *Journal of the American Veterinary Medical Association* 204 (6): 944–945.

Self, Donnie, Aleta Pierce, and John Shadduck. 1994. "A Survey of the Teaching of Ethics in Veterinary Education." *Journal of the American Veterinary Medical Association* 204 (6): 944–945.

Self, Donnie, Susan Safford, and George Shelton. 1988. "Comparison of the General Moral Reasoning of Small Animal Veterinarians vs Large Animal Veterinarians." *Journal of the American Veterinary Medical Association* 193 (12): 1509–1512.

Self, Donnie, Dawn Schrader, DeWitt Baldwin, Susan Root, Frederick Wolinsky, and John Shadduck. 1991. "Study of the Influence of Veterinary Medical Education on the Moral Development of Veterinary Students." *Journal of the American Veterinary Medical Association* 198 (5): 782–787.

Serpell, James. 2009. "Having Our Dogs and Eating Them Too: Why Animals Are a Social Issue." *Journal of Social Issues* 65 (3): 633–644.

Seymour, Jane. 2001. *Critical Moments: Death and Dying in Intensive Care*. Buckingham, PA: Open University Press.

Shaffir, William, and Robert Stebbins. 1991. *Experiencing Fieldwork: An Inside View of Qualitative Research*. New York: St. Martin's Press.

Sharp, Robert. 2005. *No Dogs in Heaven? Scenes from the Life of a Country Veterinarian.* Philadelphia: Running Press.

Shaw, Jane, Cindy Adams, and Brenda Bonnett. 2004. "What Can Veterinarians Learn from Studies of Physician-Patient Communication about Veterinarian-Client-Patient Communication?" *Journal of the American Veterinary Medical Association* 224 (5): 676–684.

Shaw, Jane, Cindy Adams, Brenda Bonnett, Susan Larson, and Debra Roter. 2008. "Veterinarian-Client-Patient Communication during Wellness Appointments versus Appointments Related to a Health Problem in Companion Animal Practice." *Journal of the American Veterinary Medical Association* 233 (10): 1576–1586.

Shaw, Jane, and Laurel Lagoni. 2007. "End-of-Life Communication in Veterinary Medicine: Delivering Bad News and Euthanasia Decision Making." *Veterinary Clinics of North America: Small Animal Practice* 37 (1): 95–108.

Slater, Margaret, and Miriam Slater. 2000. "Women in Veterinary Medicine." *Journal of the American Medical Association* 217 (4): 472–476.

Smith, Allen, and Sherryl Kleinman. 1989. "Managing Emotions in Medical School: Student Contacts with the Living and the Dead." *Social Psychology Quarterly* 52 (1): 56–69.

Smith, Carin. 2002. "Gender and Work: What Veterinarians Can Learn from Research about Women, Men, and Work." *Journal of the American Veterinary Medical Association* 220 (9): 1304–1311.

Steinhauser, Karen, Nicholas Christakis, Elizabeth Clipp, Maya McNeilly, Lauren McIntyre, and James Tulsky. 2000. "Factors Considered Important at the End of Life by Patients, Family, Physicians, and Other Care Providers." *Journal of the American Medical Association* 284 (19): 2476–2482.

Stenross, Barbara, and Sherryl Kleinman. 1989. "The Highs and Lows of Emotional Labor: Detectives' Encounters with Criminals and Victims." *Journal of Contemporary Ethnography* 17 (4): 435–452.

Stephens, Debra, and Ronald Hill. 1996. "The Loss of Animal Companions: A Humanistic and Consumption Perspective." *Society and Animals* 4 (2): 189–210.

Stern, Michael. 1996. "Psychological Elements of Attachment to Pets and Responses to Pet Loss." *Journal of the American Veterinary Medical Association* 209 (10): 1707–1711.

Stewart, Cyrus, John Thrush, George Paulus, and Patrick Hafner. 1985. "The Elderly's Adjustment to the Loss of a Companion Animal: People-Pet Dependency." *Death Studies* 9 (5–6): 383–393.

Stewart, Mary. 1999. *Companion Animal Death: A Practical and Comprehensive Guide for Veterinary Practice.* Oxford: Butterworth-Heinemann.

Stivers, Tanya. 1998. "Prediagnostic Commentary in Veterinarian-Client Interaction." *Research on Language and Social Interaction* 31 (2): 241–277.

Stover, Robert. 1989. *Making It and Breaking It: The Fate of Public Interest Commitment during Law School.* Urbana: University of Illinois Press.

Strand, Elizabeth, Tracy Zaparanick, and James Brace. 2005. "Quality of Life and Stress Factors for Veterinary Medical Students." *Journal of Veterinary Medical Education* 32 (2): 182–192.

Sutton, Robert. 1991. "Maintaining Norms about Expressed Emotions: The Case of Bill Collectors." *Administrative Science Quarterly* 36 (2): 245–268.

Swabe, Joanna. 1994. "Preserving the Emotional Order: The Display and Management of Emotion in Veterinary Interactions." *Psychologie en Maatschappij* 68 (3): 248–260.

———. 1999. *Animals, Disease and Human Society: Human-Animal Relations and the Rise of Veterinary Medicine*. London: Routledge.

———. 2000. "Veterinary Dilemmas: Ambiguity and Ambivalence in Human-Animal Interaction." In *Companion Animals and Us: Exploring the Relationships between People and Pets*, edited by Anthony Podberscek, Elizabeth Paul, and James Serpell, 292–313. New York: Cambridge University Press

Tannenbaum, Jerrold. 1985. "Ethics and Human-Companion Animal Interaction: A Plea for a Veterinary Ethics of the Human-Companion Animal Bond." *Veterinary Clinics of North America: Small Animal Practice* 15 (2): 431–447.

———. 1993. "Veterinary Medical Ethics: A Focus of Conflicting Interests." *Journal of Social Issues* 49 (1): 143–156.

———. 1995. *Veterinary Ethics: Animal Welfare, Client Relations, Competition and Collegiality*. 2nd ed. St. Louis, MO: Mosby.

Taylor, Steven, and Robert Bogdan. 1998. *Introduction to Qualitative Research Methods*. 3rd ed. New York: Wiley.

Thoits, Peggy. 1996. "Managing the Emotions of Others." *Symbolic Interaction* 19 (2): 85–110.

Timmermans, Stefan. 1999. *Sudden Death and the Myth of CPR*. Philadelphia: Temple University Press.

———. 2002. "Cause of Death vs. Gift of Life: Maintaining Jurisdiction in Death Investigation." *Sociology of Health and Illness* 24 (5): 550–574.

Tinga, Carol, Cindy Adams, Brenda Bonnett, and Carl Ribble. 2001. "Survey of Veterinary Technical and Professional Skills in Students and Recent Graduates of a Veterinary College." *Journal of the American Veterinary Medical Association* 219 (7): 924–931.

Tope, Daniel, Lindsey Chamberlain, Martha Crowley, and Randy Hodson. 2005. "The Benefits of Being There: Evidence from the Literature on Work." *Journal of Contemporary Ethnography* 34 (4): 470–493.

Tracy, Sarah, Karen Myers, and Clifton Scott. 2006. "Cracking Jokes and Crafting Selves: Sensemaking and Identity Management among Human Service Workers." *Communication Monographs* 73 (3): 283–308.

Turner, Ronny E., and Charles Edgley. 1976. "Death as Theater: A Dramaturgical Analysis of the American Funeral." *Sociology and Social Research* 60 (4): 377–392.

Ulsperger, Jason, and John Paul. 2002. "The Presentation of Paradise: Impression Management and the Contemporary Nursing Home." *Qualitative Report* 7 (4). Available at http://www.nova.edu/ssss/QR/QR7-4/ulsperger.html.

Unsworth, Kerrie, Steven Rogelberg, and Daniel Bonilla. 2010. "Animal Welfare." *Canadian Veterinary Journal* 51 (7): 775–777.

VanMaanen, John. 1988. *Tales of the Field: On Writing Ethnography*. Chicago: University of Chicago Press.

Voith, Victoria. 1985. "Attachment of People to Companion Animals." *Veterinary Clinics of North America: Small Animal Practice* 15 (2): 289–296.

Wanzer, Melissa, Melanie Booth-Butterfield, and Steve Booth-Butterfield. 2005. "If We Didn't Use Humor, We'd Cry: Humorous Coping Communication in Health Care Settings." *Journal of Health Communication* 10:105–125.

Warren, Carol, and Tracy Karner. 2005. *Discovering Qualitative Methods: Field Research, Interviews, and Analysis*. Los Angeles: Roxbury.

Watson, Katie. 2011. "Gallows Humor in Medicine." *Hastings Center Report* 41 (5): 37–45.

Wear, Delese. 1989. "Cadaver Talk: Medical Students' Accounts of Their Year-Long Experience." *Death Studies* 13: 379–391.

Wear, Delese, Julie Aultman, Joseph Varley, and Joseph Zarconi. 2006. "Making Fun of Patients: Medical Students' Perceptions and Use of Derogatory and Cynical Humor in Clinical Settings." *Academic Medicine* 81 (5): 454–462.

Weirich, Walter. 1988. "Client Grief following Pet Loss: Implication for Veterinary School Education." In *Euthanasia of the Companion Animal*, edited by William Kay, Susan Cohen, Carole Fudin, Austin Kutscher, Herbert Neiburg, Ross Grey, and Mohamed Osman, 208–212. Philadelphia: Charles Press.

Weisman, Avery. 1991. "Bereavement and Companion Animals." *Omega—Journal of Death and Dying* 22 (4): 241–248.

Wensley, Sean. 2008. "Animal Welfare and the Human-Animal Bond: Considerations for Veterinary Faculty, Students, and Practitioners." *Journal of Veterinary Medical Education* 35 (4): 532–539.

White, Debra, and Ruth Shawhan. 1996. "Emotional Responses of Animal Shelter Workers to Euthanasia." *Journal of the American Veterinary Medical Association* 280 (6): 846–849.

Wilkie, Rhoda. 2010. *Livestock/Deadstock: Working with Farm Animals from Birth to Slaughter*. Philadelphia: Temple University Press.

Williams, Sandy, Pauline Arnold, and Jennifer Mills. 2005. "Coping with Stress: A Survey of Murdoch University Veterinary Students." *Journal of Veterinary Medical Education* 32 (2): 201–212.

Williams, Sandy, and Jennifer Mills. 2000. "Understanding and Responding to Grief in Companion Animal Practice." *Australian Veterinary Practitioner* 30 (2): 55–62.

Williams, Susan, Carolyn Butler, and Mary-Ann Sontag. 1999. "Perceptions of Fourth-Year Veterinary Students about the Human-Animal Bond in Veterinary Practice and in Veterinary College Curricula." *Journal of the American Veterinary Medical Association* 215 (10): 1428–1432.

Wippen, Deborah, and George Canellos. 1991. "Burnout Syndrome in the Practice of Oncology: Result of a Random Survey of 1000 Oncologists." *Journal of Clinical Oncology* 9 (10): 1916–1920.

Witiak, Gene. 2004. *True Confessions of a Veterinarian: An Unconditional Love Story*. Centennial, CO: Glenbridge.

Wojciechowska, Janina, and Caroline Hewson. 2005. "Quality-of-Life Assessment in Pet Dogs." *Journal of the American Veterinary Medical Association* 226 (5): 722–728.

Wolfle, Thomas. 1985. "Laboratory Animal Technicians: Their Role in Stress Reduction and Human-Companion Animal Bonding." *Veterinary Clinics of North America: Small Animal Practice* 15 (2): 449–454.

Wolkomir, Michelle, and Jennifer Powers. 2007. "Helping Women and Protecting the Self: The Challenge of Emotional Labor in an Abortion Clinic." *Qualitative Sociology* 30 (2): 153–169.

Wrobel, Thomas, and Amanda Dye. 2003. "Grieving Pet Death: Normative, Gender, and Attachment Issues." *Omega—Journal of Death and Dying* 47 (4): 385–393.

Yeates, James, and David Main. 2010. "The Ethics of Influencing Clients." *Journal of the American Veterinary Medical Association* 237 (3): 263–267.

Yedidia, Michael, Colleen Gillespie, Elizabeth Kachur, Mark Schwartz, Judith Ockene, Amy Chepaitis, Clint Snyder, Aaron Lazare, and Mack Lipkin. 2003. "Effect of Communication Training on Medical Student Performance." *Journal of the American Medical Association* 290 (9): 1157–1165.

Young, Thomas R. 1990. *The Drama of Social Life: Essays in Post-Modern Social Psychology*. New Brunswick, NJ: Transaction.

Younker, Lucas, and John Fried. 1976. *Animal Doctor: The Making of a Veterinarian*. New York: E. P. Dutton.

Zeglen, Marie. 1980. "An Analysis of the 1979 Annual Survey of Graduating Veterinary Students at US and Canadian Colleges." *Journal of Veterinary Medical Education* 7: 166–175.

Zekoff, Zeke, and Karen Felsted. 2004. "Caught in the Middle: Business vs. Compassion." *Veterinary Economics*, June, 25–39.

Zussman, Robert. 1992. *Intensive Care: Medical Ethics and the Medical Profession*. Chicago: University of Chicago Press.

———. 1997. "Sociological Perspectives on Medical Ethics and Decision-Making." *Annual Review of Sociology* 23 (1): 171–189.

Index

Patricia Morris is Assistant Professor of Sociology at Drury University.